HERBAL HEALTH SECRETS
FROM EUROPE AND AROUND THE WORLD

Herbal Health Secrets from Europe and Around the World

RICHARD M. LUCAS

Parker Publishing Company, Inc.
West Nyack, New York

10 9 8 7

Library of Congress Cataloging in Publication Data

Lucas, Richard Melvin
  Herbal health secrets from Europe and around the
world.

  Includes bibliographical references.
  1. Materia medica, Vegetable. 2. Therapeutics—Pop-
ular works. I. Title.
RS164.L784 1983   615'.321   83-556
ISBN 0-13-387423-0
ISBN 0-13-387415-X {PBK}

Printed in the United States of America

Introduction

There is a growing volume of evidence indicating that various herbs used in many countries of the world are remarkably effective healing agents. For example, it was recently reported that of all remedies prescribed in the Soviet Union for the prevention and treatment of heart and vascular disease, 77% were herbal; botanical expectorants accounted for 73% of prescriptions for bronchitis and coughs; herbal remedies amounted to 74% of all medicaments given for liver and digestive troubles; and herbs accounted for 80% of the remedies taken for women's ailments.

Another of many examples is the marked interest being shown in traditional Chinese medicine. A British medical team spent eight months in China to observe Oriental healing techniques and methods. Dr. Anna Cummings, Research Associate of the University of London School of Medicine, said: "The Chinese have great respect for what they call the 'wisdom of the ancients.' Instead of dismissing everything out of the past as superstitious nonsense as we tend to do in the West, they study ancient theories with keen interest and try to develop modern techniques for applying them. The results are nothing short of miraculous."

The highly trained British medics spoke with awe about Chinese remedies which are derived from ancient herbs, roots, and barks. "They have frightfully modern pharmacies," Dr. Cummings stated, "with white-coated efficient technicians who go through these old remedies with fine-tooth combs, finding out what's in them, and then working out modern recipes that duplicate and surpass the old remedies. Their achievements in this area are absolutely remarkable."

Seven to eight hundred different kinds of herbs are exported from China to other countries, and more than 1,500 herbs plus over one thousand patent herbal remedies are used in that nation.

In America, Europe, China, Russia, South America, and other lands, thinking men and women are finding their way back to abundant health through natural plant medicine. Now, here in this book, you have a large selection of herbal recipes gathered from many parts of the world, for coping with a wide range of ailments. Along with ample coverage of herb remedies that can be easily prepared right in your own home, this book contains information on herbal products that are sold on the market in the form of extracts, tinctures, ointments, and so on. Most health food stores carry a good selection of herbs and herbal products, but if your local store cannot provide them, you can write to the mail-order firms I've listed for your convenience at the end of this book.

In one chapter you'll read about a remarkable natural healing substance found to be medicinally effective for a number of different ailments such as influenza, diseases of the sinuses and upper part of the respiratory tract, some types of hearing defects, various skin disorders, and other conditions. One doctor who prescribed this natural substance for many of his patients found that when taken regularly it creates an antibiotic disease-fighting reaction to almost any illness, without side effects.

In another chapter you'll learn of an herbal product that has been scientifically tested and proved to have an anti-stress effect. The preparation helped people cope better under the ordinary stress and tension of everyday living; counteracted threats in typical stress-induced illnesses; produced a soothing and calming effect on people who had endured months of pressure and tension; eased the strain of business and sports competition; delivered a protective effect against the stress of accidents, certain chemical toxins, radiation, and more.

Other chapters in this book cover additional ailments, such as stomach problems, insomnia, circulatory disorders, liver trouble, headaches, bowel ailments, eye afflictions, and many other disorders. And you'll find impressive case histories presented where people obtained remarkable results from the use of a harmless herb remedy. Consider the following, which are just a few of numerous examples:

• A reflex therapist wrote: "I personally know of several people who were troubled with gravel and with stones (kidney, gall bladder, and so on), and after using a Chinese herb compound they have had almost immediate relief with no recurrence of pain or distress. One man was in pain daily and had relief the day he took one set of the teas. Several months later he said he still had no further trouble.

"One interesting thing about this Chinese herb compound is that it does not have to be used for a long period of time to get results. In every case I know of, it has taken only one or two applications of the herb compound to get results."

• One woman stated that she took estrogen for more than a year to control the unpleasant symptoms of the menopause. She then switched to a harmless herb remedy, and after she had taken it for some time all symptoms of the menopause vanished and she no longer needed the estrogen.

• A researcher tested an herbal product for hemorrhoid conditions. Of 35 cases treated, most reported relief from pain, swelling, and itching, and many long-time sufferers were reportedly cured.

• One man suffered from enlarged prostate gland with complete stoppage of urine, which necessitated the use of a catheter. He says that after taking a compound herb tea he could urinate freely without using the catheter, and that the beneficial results were not temporary, but lasting.

• A doctor experienced attacks of diarrhea every time she ate. Her condition became normal after taking an herb remedy three times daily for three days.

• For ten years, Mrs. C.C. was troubled with stubborn constipation. She tried many different drug store remedies but all of them caused griping pains, loose watery bowel movements, or both. Then she began using a natural herb tea, and reported: "The bowel movements are now perfectly normal, and no griping pains."

• One woman suffered torturous migraine headaches for years. One day she learned of a simple herb tea and decided to try it. As a result, the migraine pains left and have not recurred.

• A doctor became ill with subacute colitis, symptomized by diarrhea and colic pains. He soon became completely well after taking an herbal remedy three times daily.

• Seventeen patients with ulcer of the stomach and first part of the intestine were given a natural plant remedy as the only treatment for this condition. Of the 17 who were treated, 14 obtained immediate relief from their symptoms. One patient had no relief for three days after using the remedy, but on the fifth day his symptoms disappeared.

You will find that the majority of chapters in this book include listings of several different herb remedies for each particular ailment cited. What this means to you is that since one specific remedy will not work for everyone (there are too many individual differences, too many variables), you may select one of the herbs or herb products most appropriate to your needs, and if, after giving it a sufficient trial, you find it does not help, you can switch to another. This procedure increases your chances of finding a remedy that will work for you.

In closing, I wish to point out what I have said in my previous health books. I do not prescribe. As an author and reporter, I simply pass on to you the findings and experiences of many people who have used natural herb remedies with various degrees of success.

Richard Lucas

Table of Contents

HERBAL HEALTH SECRETS
FROM EUROPE AND AROUND THE WORLD

CHAPTER 1

Herbs for the Relief of Headaches and Insomnia

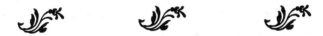

If you have a headache and don't want to take aspirin because it upsets your stomach, or if you have insomnia and want to avoid using sleeping pills, what can you do? There is a simple answer: try the remedies provided by the plant kingdom. The long history of these natural aids shows they have consistently been credited with eliminating insomnia and relieving many forms of headache pain.

BORAGE

Botanical Name: *Borago officinalis*
Common Names: Borage, Herb of Gladness

Borage is an attractive plant with lovely blue or purplish star-like flowers. In Wales it is called the "Herb of Gladness," as its use is said to cheer the spirits and overcome depression. Gerard, an early herbalist, declared that the people of his time used borage flowers to "exhilarate and make glad the mind." Bacon wrote that the herb had the power to dispel melancholia.

Borage Wine

Borage steeped in wine is an excellent remedy for insomnia.

If the herb wine is taken for a few nights, the pattern of sleeplessness is usually broken, and the remedy can be discontinued.

Borage wine is prepared as follows: Put ½ bottle of sherry and an equal amount of water in a stainless steel pot. Bring to a boil. Add 4 tablespoonfuls of borage herb, cover, and remove from the burner. Let stand until cool, then strain and pour into the sherry bottle (if it is now empty). Cap and place in the refrigerator until needed. Dose, one or two wineglassfuls. This is taken the very last thing at night, just before retiring.

Case History

D. S. relates: "When my wife and I were in our late twenties, we both had a bad siege of insomnia. We had three small children, we were working too hard, and we had many problems and worries, all of which tended to keep us keyed up. Exhausted though we were, it seemed to take hours each night before we could fall asleep. Finally I mentioned my problem to my older sister, who was interested in herbs. She made up a bottle of borage wine and told us to take a glassful at night when ready for bed. My wife and I both thought it wouldn't work, but we each drank a large glassful before putting the light out. Soon we began to relax, and the next thing we knew it was morning and the alarm clock was ringing! Ever since then we have kept a bottle of borage wine made up, ready in the refrigerator, in case we need it for a good night's sleep."

GUARANA

Botanical Name: *Paullinia cupana*
Common Names: Brazilian Cocoa, Guarana Bread

This plant is native to South America. It is often called Brazilian cocoa because the flavor of beverages made from the plant is remarkably similar to that of ordinary cocoa.

The Maues and Murdurow Indians are able to travel through jungles and across mountains for miles at a steady pace, with a stick of guarana as their only food. The sticks look like licorice, and the Indians scrape off a handful of fragments which they chew and swallow.

Guarana is classified as nutritive, stimulant, and tonic. According to South American legend, its nutritious and stimulating qualities were first discovered by the Incas three centuries before the white man first set foot on the western hemisphere.

A tea-like beverage is made from guarana by mixing about ½ teaspoonful of guarana powder in a cup of hot water. The Brazilians drink this as a refreshing and stimulating beverage, and as a remedy for headaches resulting from dissipation or depression. Its chief use in Europe and America is for relieving headaches. Dr. Wood refers to guarana as follows:

"This is an excellent remedy for sick headache. . . . Dose of the fluid extract, from ten drops to a teaspoonful. In headache, the dose may be repeated every half-hour, until the pain ceases, though one dose is often sufficient. Professor Bundy of the California Medical College says, 'When you have the headache, don't forget to take guarana.' It is a favorite remedy, and he regards it as almost sure to relieve most forms of headache. Dose of the solid extract, from one to five grains; of the sugar-coated pills, from one to two, three times a day."

It is interesting to point out that Dr. Eichenlaub, an American physician, recommends coffee for the relief of severe headaches. Guarana contains more caffeine than coffee. The caffeine content may explain the effectiveness of guarana as a headache remedy.

Guarana, of course, should be avoided where the drinking of coffee or tea is forbidden.

MARJORAM

Botanical Name: *Origanum vulgare*
Common Name: Wild Marjoram

Marjoram is a perennial herb that grows freely in many parts of the world. The botanical name, Origanum, is taken from two Greek words, *oros* (mountain) and *ganos* (joy), because of the lovely appearance these plants give to the mountains and hillsides on which they grow.

For ages, the herb has been used in food and as a folk remedy. It was also a custom in early Greece and Rome to prepare wreaths from the leaves, with which to crown young married couples, as the plant was believed to have been sown by the goddess Venus. In India, marjoram was regarded as a sacred herb.

Modern Uses

Marjoram has a fragrant, balsamic odor, and warm aromatic taste, both of which properties are preserved when the herb is dried. An infusion of the plant is used to relieve headache, nervous insomnia, and indigestion.

A correspondent writes: "I was looking for something that would help me sleep nights and this I found among the pages of old almanacs. 'Take a half-teaspoon of marjoram in one cup of hot milk at bedtime. It is very soothing.' Here I have had marjoram in the house for some time and didn't know what it was for. Have been taking it for some time and find it so wonderful; I can now enjoy a good night's rest."

ALMONDS

Botanical Name: *Amygdalus communis*
Common Name: Sweet Almond

The almond tree is native to the warmer areas of western Asia and North Africa, but it has been cultivated in many parts of the world.

Modern researchers have discovered that almonds contain salicylates, an effective pain-killing agent. Salicylates are also contained in aspirin, but there they are chemically synthesized, whereas those in almonds are natural.

According to Dr. Ivan Danhof, if you were to chew four or five almonds you would get the same amount of salicylates as you would from an average size aspirin tablet. And if you took more than 10 or 12, you'd get a fair amount of salicylate which would be absorbed into the blood, and could give the same kind of relief from headache pain that you'd get with taking aspirin tablets. However, it takes longer to relieve a headache through the use of almonds than it does with aspirin.

Dr. Danhof explains that almonds could be a possible alternative to aspirin, as there are many people who take large amounts of aspirin, and as a result suffer distress of their stomach lining.

PASSION FLOWER

Botanical Name: *Passiflora incarnata*
Common Names: Passion Vine, Granadilla

Passion flower is a handsome climber and is regarded as one of the most graceful and lovely plants that can be used for covering trellises and arbors. There are many species, but most are native to the West Indies and the southern part of the United States. In their native habitat they often climb to the top of the highest trees where they sustain themselves by means of tendrils, and send out an abundance of beautiful white and purple flowers. The Spanish friars in America were the first to call this flower the "flower of passion" as they saw in it a symbolic representation of some of the objects associated with the crucifixion.

Remedial Uses of Passion Flower

Passion flower was an ancient herbal sedative, antispasmodic, and nervine, and is still used as such in various countries of the world today. Dr. Leclerc of Paris found that it had a calming effect on nervous restlessness and insomnia. Many years of experience showed that its use resulted in neither disorientation nor depression.

Dr. Eric Powell describes passion flower as the remedy that brings peace to mind and body. He says: "Acting through the brain and nervous system it relaxes where there is muscular or organic tension, eases pain (pain is always associated with tension and contraction), and promotes a state of calmness throughout the entire organism."

For sleepless nights, T. C. Taws, Medical Herbalist of England, advises a mixture of one-half ounce each of passion flower, valerian, and hops added to one pint of boiling water. The container is immediately removed from the burner and the tea allowed to stand for a few hours. "Strain, then take a wineglassful half an hour before retiring."

For insomnia, Dr. Clymer recommends combining one ounce tincture of passion flower with one ounce tincture of scullcap herb. The dose is 20 to 60 drops in a small glass of water.

FEVERFEW

Botanical Name: *Chrysanthemum parthenium*
Common Name: Featherfoil, Featherfew

This plant grows abundantly in fields and waysides. It belongs to the chamomile family and contains similar therapeutic properties, though in a lesser degree.

In Finland, feverfew is used as a nerve tonic. The Germans employ it for hysterical complaints, headaches, nervousness, and depression. The tea is prepared as an infusion by placing a heaping teaspoon of the herb in a cup and adding boiling water. This is allowed to stand until cold, then strained. One cup of the cold tea is taken two or three times a day, a good mouthful at a time.

An Interesting Case

In an early British herbal, Sir John Hill wrote: "The mother of the late Sir William Bowyer told me that during the first half of her life, she suffered from terrible and constant headaches, fixed in one small spot of the cranium, raging to distraction." He went on to say that a maidservant cured her with feverfew tea, a quart of boiling water poured on two handfuls of the flowers and leaves.

WILLOW

Botanical Name: *Salix alba*
Common Names: European Willow, White Willow

This well-known tree is indigenous to Europe but has been naturalized in North America. There are many varieties of willow, and most are valued for their pain-relieving and fever-reducing properties.

In herbal medicine, the willow is classed as anodyne, diaphoretic, febrifuge, tonic, antiseptic, and astringent. This tree has often been cited as one of nature's greatest gifts to man because its bark contains the glucoside *salicin*, an effective pain killer.

The American Indians were well acquainted with the remedial power of the willows. The bark, prepared as a tea, was used for many purposes, but especially to reduce fever and to ease the pains of headache and rheumatism.

Modern Uses

Willow bark tea is still used as a natural pain reliever. It is considered a valuable domestic remedy for headaches, especially those resulting from colds. The tea is prepared by slowly boiling two ounces of the cut bark in two pints of water for 15 minutes. The decoction is then strained, and one teacupful is taken four or five times a day.

Another method that may be used calls for soaking one or two teaspoons of the cut bark in a large cup of cold water for four hours. It is then brought to a boil for three minutes, after which it is strained. One cup is taken daily, a large mouthful at a time.

LIME FLOWERS

Botanical Name: *Tilia europaea*
Common Names: Lindenflowers, Linden Tree

This is a large tree with yellowish-white fragrant flowers that hang in clusters. Honey made from the flowers is considered the most flavorful in the world and is used extensively in medicine and liqueurs.

The Germans were especially fond of the Linden tree and named one of their Berlin streets "Unter den Linden" (under the Linden).

The fragrance of lime flowers has a soothing and relaxing effect. It is claimed that even sitting under a lime tree in bloom causes drowsiness.

Dr. T. H. Bartram, an English medical herbalist, says: "If you are a victim of agryphiaphobia, which is just another word for saying you can't sleep o' nights, a cup of lime tea can relax blood vessels of the brain and reduce tension. Good to take at bedtime to induce sleep."

Lime flowers are used in the form of an infusion. One teaspoonful is placed in a cup and boiling water poured over. The cup is covered with a saucer and the tea allowed to stand for 15 minutes, then strained. One teaspoonful of honey is added and the beverage taken warm, just before bedtime.

FRINGE TREE

Botanical Name: *Chionanthus virginica*
Common Names: Snowdrop Tree, Old Man's Beard

Fringe tree is considered an exceptionally valuable remedy for "liverish" or bilious migraine headache. Refer to the chapter on the liver.

CHAMOMILE

Botanical Name: *Matricaria chamomilla*
Common Names: German Chamomile, Single Chamomile

The flower heads of German chamomile are much smaller

than those of the Roman variety. This European plant has also been naturalized in the United States. The flower is said to be dedicated to St. Anne, the Mother of the Virgin, seemingly because of the herb's botanical name *Matricaria*, which is derived from *mater* and *cara*, meaning "beloved mother."

German chamomile tea is used as a sedative, tonic, and carminative. It is a popular beverage in European countries where it is taken before retiring to assure a good night's sleep. It is also reputed to be a valuable children's remedy, especially for the treatment of nightmare and restless sleep. An old English physician, Dr. Schall, claimed that the tea was not only an effective remedy for nightmare but was also an excellent preventative of this complaint.

For children, the usual infusion (prepared as ordinary tea) is taken in doses of one or two tablespoonfuls three or four times a day; for adults, three or four cups daily.

Mrs. W. R. of London writes: "One herbal remedy we find very helpful is chamomile tea taken last thing at night. My husband grows the chamomile and I pick and dry the flower heads. The tea always gives a good night's sleep and also helps digestion."

WOOD BETONY

Botanical Name: *Betonica officinalis*
Common Name: Bishopwort

Throughout the centuries, this woodland plant was cultivated in the gardens of apothecaries and monasteries, and may still be seen growing around the sites of these ancient buildings. The name of the herb is from the Celtic *ben*, "the head," and *ton*, "good," in reference to its reputed virtues as a remedy for certain head complaints.

Records show that Antonius Musa, physician to Augustus Caesar, valued the plant as an effective remedy for many ailments, and Culpeper remarks that "it was not the practice of Caesar to keep fools about him."

Modern Uses

Dr. Evans, an English doctor, refers to the medicinal value of wood betony: "In medical practice I have found many patients suffering from nervous tension who get irritable and excited and complain of head pains of a purely functional nature. They also sleep badly, sometimes complaining of dreams. For this symptomatic picture I strongly recommend wood betony. A simple infusion can be made with one ounce of the herb to one pint of boiling water, a wineglassful to be taken frequently. I have found it highly successful and of use in domestic medicine."

SKULLCAP

Botanical Name: *Scutellaria laterifolia*
Common Names: Blue Skullcap, Hoodwort, Quaker Bonnet

This plant grows to about three feet in height and bears flowers of a pale blue color. Its natural habitat is North America, Europe, and the eastern part of Asia.

In botanic medicine the herb is considered a valuable nervine tonic and antispasmodic. Dr. Fearn refers to its use as follows: "Scutellaria, by its action through the cerebro-spinal centers, is a most valuable remedy, controlling nervous irritation, calming hysterical excitement. . . . In restlessness and excitement, with insomnia, following prolonged application to business, long sickness or physical exhaustion, it is most useful."

Combined Formulas

Skullcap is generally combined with other herbs. For example, Dr. J. R. Yemm gives the following account: "A gentleman I met recently, who appeared to be in robust health, informed me that for three years he had been continually under the treatment of various doctors for nervous debility and insomnia. Treatment which included bromides and other drugs had been of no avail. Being induced to try natural medicine, he prepared an infusion from skullcap, one ounce; hops, half-ounce; gentian root, crushed, half-ounce. After only one week of the herbal treatment he was sleeping well; at the end of two months, fully recovered."

Here is another formula that reputedly has worked well for some people. Thoroughly mix together equal parts of skullcap, catnip, and peppermint. Place one or two heaped teaspoonfuls of the mixture in a cup of boiling water. Cover the cup with a saucer and allow it to stand until lukewarm, then strain it. Take one cupful warm at night, upon retiring.

RAISINS

Miss U. M. P. of London writes: "Some readers might be interested to learn how I found chewing dried raisins very helpful in curing simple migraine. I don't think it would be very applicable in a more severe type of headache with one-sided pain. But when I get disturbed eyesight without head pain I find that chewing a few raisins clears the vision and restores steadiness in a matter of minutes. So I always carry a few with me."

VALERIAN

Botanical Name: *Valeriana officinalis*
Common Names: All Heal, English Valerian

This plant is found throughout Europe and Northern Asia. It is very common in England, where it grows in marshy thickets and on the borders of rivers.

In the Middle Ages the root was used as a medicine, a spice, and a perfume.

Valerian is a traditional remedy for functional disturbances of the nervous system, and is said to help overcome insomnia. In an article published in the *British Medical Journal* (1928), Dr. Manson wrote that valerian "was perhaps the earliest method of treating the neurosis."

Constituents of Valerian

Valerian contains valerianic, acetic, and formic acids in addition to an essential oil, resin, starch, a glucoside, and two alkaloids—chatrine and valerianine. In botanic medicine the action of the root is classified as nervine, anodyne, antispasmodic, sedative, and carminative.

Recorded Uses

Dr. Yemm refers to the value of valerian as follows: "It is soothing and diffusive, gives relief in irritability of the nervous system, insomnia, and hysteria. It exerts a marked influence on the cerebro-spinal system, acting directly on those parts, thereby causing steadiness in unbalanced conditions. The root eases pain and promotes sleep. Those suffering from overstrained nerves find it especially beneficial.

"Preparation and uses—make the infusion as follows: valerian, one ounce; water (boiling) one pint. Dose: one or two wineglassfuls four times daily."

Herbalists often combine valerian with two or more suitable plants. Here is a popular formula for insomnia, nervous tension, and restlessness: Mix 1 tablespoon valerian, 1 tablespoon skullcap, 1 tablespoon catnip, and 1 tablespoon celery seeds. Prepare as an infusion with one pint of boiling water. Cover and allow to steep for ten minutes, then strain. Herbalists recommend one cup of the hot tea three or four times a day. Sip the beverage slowly.

HONEY

Many people troubled with insomnia have found that one or two teaspoons of honey stirred in a cup of warm milk is a remarkably effective nightcap.

VIOLET

Botanical Name: *Viola odorata*
Common Names: Sweet Violet, Blue Violet

The common sweet violet, grown extensively in gardens, figures prominently in European literature and even entered the political field of Napoleon's time. It was said to be the secret badge of his adherents during his absence.

The violet was a favorite of both the Romans and Greeks, and was the national flower of Athens. Orators endeavoring to win the favorable attention of the people addressed them as "Athenians crowned with violets." In Persia, the Mohammedans flavored their sherbets with violets, while the Romans drank a perfumed wine made from the blossoms. It was also considered a love potion.

In the symbolic language of flowers, faithfulness is represented by the blue variety of violets.

Remedial Use

Herbalists maintain that violet tea has been helpful in dispelling some cases of headache pain, including migraine. A handful of the dried leaves are placed in a saucepan and covered with two cupfuls of cold water. This is brought to a boil and removed upon boiling, then strained. One teacupful is taken morning and night, after meals.

VERVAIN

Botanical Name: *Verbena officinalis*
Common Names: Herb of Grace, Holy Vervain

Vervain, a perennial bearing numerous small purplish flowers, is native to Europe, China, and Japan. In the Chinese language, the plant was given two different names, Ma-pien-tsao and Lung-ya-tsao. The "Holy Vervain" or verbena has no odor, and is not to be confused with the lemon-scented verbena of our gardens.

Modern Uses

Vervain has a long-standing reputation as a remedy for relieving various types of headaches, such as mild, congestive, or nervous sick headache, caused by fatigue or tension. The Chinese have also found the herb to be helpful for chronic and migraine headaches which can sometimes be traced to female disorders such as ovarian and uterine derangement.

In reference to the value of vervain tea as a remedy for chronic headache, Dr. Bartram of England writes: "A cup of vervain tea is bringing relief to many wedded to this affliction (headache). One or two heaped teaspoonfuls of the dried herb placed in a teacup filled with boiling water and allowed to cool, should not be overlooked in a search for freedom from pain. One wineglassful of the cold infusion, or more in desperate cases, may be taken three or four times daily. It will not cure every case, but it is worth trying. It can do no harm."

The tea may also be prepared from instant vervain tea bags, or a quart of boiling water may be poured into a large bowl containing two ounces of vervain. The bowl is covered with a lid, and the tea allowed to steep until cool, then strained. The cold infusion is taken in teacupful doses throughout the day.

Case Histories

• One woman reported that for years she suffered from migraine headache which could not be cured. Then one day she read in a health publication that the use of vervain sometimes effectively relieves migraine. She said: "I insisted on trying it. After the first few cachets of dried vervain in my tea, the migraine pains left me and have not been felt since."

• Another woman who suffered periodic attacks of migraine wrote: "It was only after six years of torture that I discovered the effective relief in a simple infusion of vervain, an herb popular as a health tizane on the continent and elsewhere, which can be obtained in small cachets sufficient to make a teacupful. I took several teacupfuls daily."

SUMMARY

1. Throughout the ages, remedies from the plant kingdom have helped many people to overcome insomnia, and to relieve nagging headache pains.

2. The botanicals used in domestic medicine as sedatives and pain relievers are gentle and non-habit forming.

3. Fringe tree is considered an exceptionally valuable remedy for "liverish" or migraine headache. Refer to the chapter on the liver.

CHAPTER 2

Nature's Remedies for Liver and Gallbladder Complaints

Physicians explain that the liver, the largest gland in the human body, is made up of one million lobules, each single lobule consisting of approximately 350,000 cells. The liver is a remarkable chemical factory which detoxifies the blood. Whenever toxic substances reach the liver by means of the portal vein from the intestinal tract, they are intercepted, which protects the body from harm. An experiment was conducted by a Russian scientist in which two animals were given an equal dose of lethal poison intravenously, the first into an ordinary vein, and the second into the portal vein. The first animal died, but the second remained unaffected, as the poison was rendered harmless by the liver. It was not until the lethal dose was multiplied five times that the second animal finally died.

The Liver—Guardian of Good Health

Most of us do not realize how often the liver may have saved our lives by detoxifying deadly poisons that would otherwise pass into our blood. For we are exposed to a multitude of toxins: for example—medicinal drugs; alcohol; tobacco; various food preservatives; excessive protein intake; agricultural sprays which abound in lead, arsenic, etc.; liver-poisoning emotions such as stress, irritation, anger and frustration; pollution of the atmosphere by dust, smoke, and the fumes from automobiles, jet airplanes, and gigantic manufacturing plants. In order for the liver to eliminate various drugs and other toxins from the body, it must be as healthy as possible.

Derangement of liver function results in symptoms such as lack of energy, headaches, lassitude, general torpor, and various digestive disturbances such as flatulence, bloat, and bowel disturbances.

A Word about the Gallbladder

Bile is a yellow fluid secreted by the liver into the intestinal tract. It helps to produce an alkaline reaction in the intestines, to absorb and emulsify fats, and to prevent putrefaction. The gallbladder is a hollow pear-shaped organ which stores and concentrates bile. It is situated beneath the liver. If the bile duct does not contract enough to completely empty itself, or if the flow of bile is sluggish and thick or congested, then a host of problems can occur. Some examples are biliousness, bilious sick headache, indigestion, gas, bloating, dizziness, nausea, disturbance of vision, intolerance of fats, halitosis, jaundice, and gallstones. In chronic conditions of poor gallbladder function, the skin and the whites of the eyes may become yellowish.

Gallstones can be formed from different substances, as for example calcium phosphate or calcium carbonate, but the cholesterol type is regarded as the easiest type to dissolve. The size of the stones can vary from gravel to the size of a small plum. Sometimes a moderately large gallstone may be washed into the bile duct by a flood of gall, and becomes lodged there. It causes extreme pain, known as gallstone colic, and is often accompanied by nausea, vomiting, and cold sweating.

NATURAL REMEDIES FOR COPING WITH LIVER AND GALLBLADDER AILMENTS

DANDELION

Botanical Name: *Leontodon taraxacum*
Common Name: Priest's Crown

The common dandelion is a native of Greece. It thrives under almost any condition and has spread to nearly every part of the world. The first part of the botanical name *Leontodon* was derived from two Greek words meaning "lion" and "tooth." The word *dandelion* has a similar meaning and is a corruption of the French *dent de lion* or lion's tooth. Some believe the name was given to the plant because the jagged leaf looks like the teeth of a lion. Others claim it was because of the yellow flower which bears a resemblance to the golden teeth of the heraldic lion. The name *taraxacum* was taken from an Arabian alteration of a Greek word meaning "edible." The herb was first mentioned as a medicine in the writings of Arabian physicians in the tenth century, under the name *Tarakhshagun*.

Dandelion was also mentioned in Welsh medicines of the 13th century. The roots have long been valued as a medicine on the continent, and the plant is largely cultivated in India as a remedy for liver complaints. In France the roots are cooked as a vegetable and added to broth, and in Germany they are sliced and used in salads.

Health Properties in Dandelion

Dandelion greens contain 7,000 units of vitamin A per ounce. They also provide an abundance of vitamins B_1 and C. Two alkaloids, the more valuable of which is *taraxacin*, have been isolated from dandelion root. It also contains potash, inulin, pectin, sugar, and levulin.

In Europe, many scientific experiments conducted with the plant have confirmed the traditional belief that its use is beneficial to the health of the liver. Dr. Le Clerc and others found it to be a true hepatic stimulant. The root is said to contain more of its active principles during the autumn than at any other season of the year; however, the composition of the soil in different areas must also be taken into account.

The dandelion is a wonderful purifying agent as it contains a good assortment of alkaline salts such as calcium, sodium, and potassium. We are told that it stimulates the flow of bile as well as producing a mild action on the liver. Due to its content of potash, it is considered an effective diuretic. Dandelion also contains cholin, a factor of the vitamin B complex which science has found to be essential to liver function.

Dandelion Remedies

In olden times, herbalists who peddled their botanicals among European villages were known as Green Men, and a number of English country inns still bear this name today. Plant remedies of the Green Men were handed down from one generation to the next, and many formulas have survived to the present time.

The following herbal combination was recommended as a daily health beverage to sharpen the senses, maintain resilience of the arteries, and strengthen the liver:

Simple infusion (tea): Nettles, two oz.; dandelion, one oz.; coltsfoot, one oz. Mix. Place two or three teaspoonfuls in a teapot and infuse as ordinary tea. Add sugar and milk to taste. Drink a teacupful as a beverage instead of coffee.

Other European Dandelion Remedies

The following remedies are used in various parts of Europe:

- One ounce of dandelion roots is simmered slowly in a pint of water for 10 minutes. The tea is then strained and sweetened with honey. Several glasses are taken in the course of a day.
- Two ounces of freshly sliced dandelion root in two pints of water are boiled down to one pint, then one ounce of compound tincture of horseradish is added. The dose is from 2 to 4 ounces. Used as a domestic remedy for a sluggish state of the liver.
- One ounce dandelion root, 1 ounce black horehound herb, ½ ounce sweet flag root, ¼ ounce mountain flax. The herbs are mixed thoroughly, then simmered in 3 pints of water down to 1½ pints. A wineglassful of the strained decoction is taken after meals for biliousness.
- For conditions of gallstones, 1 ounce dandelion root, 1 ounce balm herb, 1 ounce parsley root, ½ ounce ginger root, and ½ ounce licorice root are mixed together and placed in two quarts of water. This is gently simmered down to 1 quart, then strained. One wineglassful is taken every two hours.

Dandelion Remedies of a British Medical Herbalist

T. H. Bartram, the medical herbalist of England, regards the healing virtues of the dandelion as follows:[1]

How often has a sufferer trodden underfoot leaves which might

---

[1]Health from Herbs, June 1953.

have cured his cirrhosis [hardening] of the liver and thus lengthened his life?

In an age when simplicity is crucified in the interests of complexity, it is hard for one trained along orthodox lines to perceive the subtle healing power in this lesser member of the leontodons [dandelion].

It has taken unorthodox practitioners over 50 years to convince a few genito-urinary specialists of the superiority of dandelion coffee in the prevention of gallstones in patients unduly susceptible to their formation.

Hepatitis, or inflammation of the liver, and jaundice, when uncomplicated, readily yield to the taraxacine of dandelion. Its inulin is nutritive, especially in the wasting of the anemias when liver malfunction is often a causative factor.

Methods of preparation:

Simple Decoction—Half ounce dried roots should be placed in a vessel, brought to a boil in 1 pint of water, allowed to simmer for 10 minutes, and taken in wineglassful doses after meals three times daily. Excessive boiling impairs its strength.

Fluid Extract—Dose, half-teaspoonful to a wineglass of water, after meals, three times daily.

Dandelion Coffee—Roots should be slowly roasted in an oven and pulverized by pounding in a pestle and mortar, or by grinding. Addition of a little salt improves. The result can be used with hot milk and sweetening.

NOTE: Dandelion coffee has become a commercial product which is now sold by health food stores and various herb companies.

Case History with the Use of Dandelion

Around the turn of the century, Dr. Sparks wrote: "Fifteen years ago I was afflicted with the liver complaint. I used all my skill trying to cure it but failed. I then tried two physicians, Doctors Wilson and Jordan, but without success."

Mr. Sparks goes on to say that an old nurse told him that dandelion root was an effective folk remedy for this disorder, so he decided to give it a try. He claims that its use promptly restored his health. From then on he employed the herb in his practice, regarding it as his favorite prescription for liver complaint. According to Dr. Sparks, his patients obtained favorable results, "either by the simple extract of the herb and root, or by taking a teacupful of a strong decoction of it twice a day." He adds, "In almost every instance I have succeeded in restoring those who have used this plant."

CAMOMILE

Botanical Name: *Anthemis nobilis*
Common Name: Roman Camomile

This is a European plant which grows wild in temperate regions and has been naturalized in the United States. The botanical name is from *anthemon*, "a flower," in reference to the great number of flowers the herb produces. It was given the common name of Roman camomile by Joachim Camerarius in 1598.

Camomile has an aroma similar to that of apples, a characteristic noted by the Greeks. It was because of the odor that they named the herb "ground apple"—*Kamai* (on the ground) and *melon* (an apple)—indicating the origin of the name *camomile*. In Spain it is called "Manzanilla," signifying "a little apple."

The medicinal use of Roman camomile dates from antiquity. The Egyptians consecrated it to their gods because of the high esteem in which it was held as a remedial agent. In Rome, a tea was prepared from the flowers and used as a bitter tonic and blood purifier. The French drank it after meals to aid digestion. Women used the tea to relieve menstrual cramps and suppressed menstruation. The herb was also believed to ease pain and remove fatigue when used in the bath.

Constituents and Modern Uses

Roman camomile contains volatile oil, tannic acid, anthemic acid, and a glucoside.

Among its various modern uses, camomile tea is sometimes prescribed by medical herbalists for treating the condition of gallstones. Certain dietary restrictions are also followed during the course of treatment. In one of her books, Claudia V. James of Canada says, "Taken as a tea it [camomile] dissolves gallstones . . . I can vouch for this myself." In another of her books she writes of a man who gave her a few of the gallstones he had removed by surgery. He told her, "You can't dissolve these with camomile flowers. My wife and I have been pounding them with a big hammer and we can't break them." Mrs. James replied, "Wait and see." She adds, "So I made a solution of 14 camomile flowers in a tablespoon of boiling water, poured it into a small glass, and dropped two gallstones into it. The next day they were in four pieces. In five days they were like grit, and in ten days they had disappeared altogether."

Camomile tea is prepared by placing a teaspoonful of the flowers in a teacup and adding boiling water. The cup is covered with a saucer and allowed to stand for 10 minutes, then strained. One teacupful is taken 2 or 3 times a day.

OLIVE

Botanical Name: *Olea europaea*
Common Name: Olive

The olive tree, native to the warm regions of Europe and Asia, was introduced into America around the year 1769. It is a tree of great antiquity, attaining the age of over two thousand years. It is said that eight of the original olive trees in the Garden of Gethsemane are still in existence.

In *The Stones of Venice* Ruskin says: "What the elm and the oak are to England the olive is to Italy. It has been well for painters to have seen and felt the olive tree, to have loved it for Christ's sake ... to have loved it even to the dimness of its foliage, subdued and faint of hue as if the ashes of the Gethsemane agony had been cast upon it forever."

Universal Symbol of Peace

Since time immemorial the olive tree has been regarded as a symbol of peace in almost every land in the world. Early navigators found that green olive branches carried in the hands or placed in the ground were universally employed and understood as emblems of peace among all islanders, even those of the South Seas. The Greeks prayed for prosperity and peace with green olive boughs held in their hands, garlands around their necks, and crowns upon their heads. Among the Chinese, disputes or quarrels were settled by sending the offended person an olive wrapped in red paper.

A Valuable Food Oil

The olive is one of our most valuable sources of food oil. Due to its high content of potassium, it is considered a good cleansing and healing agent. It is also rich in sodium and calcium. Olive oil is easily digested and imparts a generally soothing and healing influence to the digestive tract. Unfortunately, it is often diluted or adulterated with cottonseed oil for commercial sale. The pure or virgin olive oil is more expensive and can be easily recognized by its taste if compared with that of a preserved olive. Medicinally, the pure oil is used both internally and externally for the treatment of a variety of disorders.

Olive Oil as a Gall Bladder Tonic and Gallstone Remover

In an issue of *Minerva Dietologica*, Dr. E. Granata writes that olive oil is a valuable preventative against gallstones. The oil causes strong healthy contractions of the gallbladder, greatly favoring complete emptying, and thus can be regarded as a very good gallbladder tonic. Dr. Granata's findings were confirmed by an International News Service release in which it was reported that olive oil is an essential factor in stimulating bile secretion and absorbing fatty acids.

Olive oil has been known to remove small gallstones, but should not be used if an X-ray reveals a large stone as it may become lodged in the bile duct. There are different versions of using the oil. Dr. Eric Powell of England recommends the following:

"One half-pint of best olive oil and the juice of six lemons are required. Take a moderate dose of Epsom salts and one hour later take a small wineglass of oil followed immediately by a drink of lemon juice. Repeat the dose in five minutes, and take more lemon juice. The lemon juice may be taken raw or very slightly diluted. It is better used undiluted. The lemon prevents nausea and vomiting, especially with those who find it difficult to take oil of any nature. Later in the day another dose of Epsom salts may be taken if there has not been a bowel movement."

Another version suggests mixing thoroughly ½ cup of olive oil with ½ cup of fresh grapefruit or lemon juice, and drinking the mixture at bedtime. In the morning a cup of hot water is taken.

Dr. Vogel of Switzerland presents the following:[2]

If one aims at the removal of gallstones, the treatment to accomplish it is not a simple matter. I recall an Italian lady who consulted me in connection with an operation she was advised to undergo for the purpose of removing her gallstones. Her family doctor, who discovered them, urged for immediate surgical intervention, but the patient was obviously scared stiff and determined to try and find some other, less radical method of removing them.

---

[2]The *Liver*, Bioforce Verlag (AR), Switzerland, 1962, pp. 94–5.

As I know full well that Italians have no difficulty in swallowing oil, I recommended the oil cure. For that purpose, the intestinal tract has to be thoroughly cleansed, preferably by means of soaked prunes or figs, or freshly milled linseeds. If that is not sufficient, an enema can be taken in addition. When the colon is empty, from 4 to 14 fluid ounces of oil should be swallowed. One then lies down, turns over on to one's right side and remains in that position for two hours. Well, the lady returned a few days after the treatment had been performed and, seeing her beaming face, I knew at once that it had been a success; a lot of stones came away the morning after she had taken the oil, and an X-ray confirmed that an operation had become unnecessary, because there were no longer any stones in the gallbladder. The lady's doctor could hardly believe it, but it's no use quarrelling with an X-ray, is it? Quite naturally, not every oil cure achieves such wonderful results, for there are not many people who can take a pint of oil—as that lady did! One then has to compromise, take less oil and also spread it over a few days. This will still bring away the smaller stones, also purify the liver and, above all, the gallbladder so that any trouble that might arise from the larger remaining stones will probably be kept at bay for some time. An old, chronic disorder that suddenly becomes acute again and is accompanied by high fever and an increase in white blood cells would, however, suggest a suppurative inflammation which only the surgeon can deal with.

FRINGE TREE

Botanical Name: *Chionanthus virginica*
Common Name: Snowdrop Tree, Old Man's Beard

Fringe tree is an ornamental shrub, easily cultivated and especially adapted to lawns because of its beautiful flowers and deep green, glossy foliage. The botanical name is from *chion*, "snow," and *anthos*, "a flower," in reference to its long racemes of pure white flowers.

The healing virtues of fringe tree were well known to the American Indians and early colonists. Frontier doctors boiled a tea from the bark and employed it for headaches of a bilious character.

In modern herbal medicine the rootbark of fringe tree is employed as a remedy for such conditions as acute jaundice, enlarged spleen, and weakness of the liver. It also reportedly liquidifes the bile and helps to prevent the formation of gallstones. In addition, it is regarded among herbalists and home-opaths as a valuable remedy for bilious sick headache (migraine).

Dr. Felter of Lloyd's reported the following information on fringe tree:

> Chionanthus exerts a special influence upon the liver, and to a slight extent upon all the organs engaged in digestion. The indications for its exhibition are: yellowness of the skin and eyes; slight or fully developed jaundice, with a sense of uneasiness and general pains simulating colic. It is one of the most certain remedies employed, whether the case is of jaundice, formation and passage of gallstone, bilious colic (indicated by yellowness of skin), acute dyspepsia, acute or chronic inflammation of the liver, or the irritable liver of the hard drinker.
>
> Chionanthus is also indicated by a sallow skin, with expressionless eyes and hepatic tenderness; the passage of light grayish stools and scant urine which stains the clothing yellow. The liver pain may range from a slight uneasiness, with a feeling of weight and fullness, to an intense pain converging from the gallbladder to the umbilicus, and attended with nausea, vomiting, and marked prostration.

General Directions

The tea is prepared with one ounce of the cut bark of fringe tree to one pint of boiling water. This is simmered very slowly for ten minutes, then strained. One wineglassful is taken three times daily. Of the fluid extract, one-half to one teaspoonful in a little water should be taken two or three times daily.

Interesting Case History

Early in the century, Professor I.J.M. Goss wrote:

> Some thirty-two years ago, I had been very badly salivated in an attack of bilious fever, by my preceptor, and it resulted in an attack of jaundice, for which I was again salivated several times, with the result of an increase of the jaundice. I now gave up to die, for I had tried six or eight of the best physicians of Georgia. Their remedies were the same, which only increased the disease. So I had, after trying the remedies for four or five months, given up in despair. About this time I was induced by a fellow-student to try the "old woman's remedy," Chionanthus (Old Man's Gray Beard, as they called it), which grew plentifully upon the sandy land near Augusta, Georgia, where I was then attending lectures,

and as the faculty had utterly failed to cure, or even benefit me, I concluded to try it.

I procured a small quantity, and made a tincture in gin, and took a tablespoonful before each meal. In a few days my appetite began to improve, and my skin very rapidly cleared, and in some ten days my jaundice was gone; my skin was clear of bilious hue, and I felt like another man. I subsequently met with many cases of jaundice, and found the remedy so prompt to remove it that I published my experience in the *Eclectic Medical Journal* of Philadelphia, since which time I have used it in a great many cases with success. I now use a saturated tincture. Dose of the tincture, one drachm [approx. 1 teaspoonful] three times a day.

"Liverish" (Migraine) Headache

Some authorities maintain that liver trouble is one of the most common among the many causes of migraine headache, due to a back-up of bile into the bloodstream. Once the thickened bile starts to flow, the nauseated, "liverish" sufferer begins to vomit the greenish-yellow bile, sometimes every several hours both day and night, often for two or three days. When at long last the excess bile is completely eliminated, the headache is finally relieved. But as long as the backed-up bile is retained in the system, the nausea and blinding headache persist. Therefore, to get the bile flowing as soon as possible during an attack, Chinese herbalists advise the sufferer to drink one or two glasses of plain hot water. Drinking the water usually starts an amount of the bile flowing, which can then be eliminated through vomiting. The glasses of hot water are continued every hour or two as needed, until the excess bile is completely eliminated. This means of washing out the bile from the system shortens the duration of the attack and more quickly relieves the blinding migraine headaches.

Although the hot water treatment may bring prompt relief during a spell of liverish migraine, it will not cure the condition. That is, it will not prevent future attacks from occurring. Therefore, the real aim is to heal the ailment and produce lasting results. Following are examples of fringe tree remedies used in Chinese medicine, which have reputedly proved helpful in a number of cases of liverish migraine.

1. One-half ounce each of fringe tree, dandelion root, vervain, ginger root, motherwort, marshmallow root, wild

carrot (Daucus carota), and centaury (*Erythraea cen-taurium*) are mixed together and simmered in one quart of boiling water for 15 minutes in a covered vessel. The decoction is strained and one teacupful is taken three times daily before meals. This formula is taken for several weeks, or longer if necessary, because the effects are reputedly slow and gradual. It is said that the period between the migraine attacks should lengthen, and the severity of the attacks should lessen.

2. Twelve drops of the fluid extract of fringe tree are taken in a little warm water, three times a day after meals.

3. The fluid extract of fringe tree combined with the fluid extract of an herb known as Greater Celandine (*Chelidonium majus*) is another remedy which has reportedly brought relief to sufferers of liverish migraine. Equal amounts of the two fluid extracts are mixed together, and one teaspoonful in a little warm water is taken three times daily after meals. In some instances this combination has also been known to dissolve gallstones, when the treatment is continued long enough.

Important Dietary Tips for Liverish Migraine

In addition to the use of the herb remedies for liverish migraine, the Chinese advise sufferers to avoid eating or drinking anything cold. All foods or fluids should be warm or hot. It is also claimed that victims of this type of chronic migraine headache are sensitive to external cold as well as internal cold. Therefore, the body should never be permitted to become chilled, especially in the upper abdomen and waist areas. In cold weather, extra warm clothing should be worn around the bodily areas mentioned, and any exposure to strong winds should be avoided at all times.

Fried foods, pastries, gravies, and dairy products such as milk, cream, eggs, and cheese are to be omitted from the diet. If the person is troubled with irregularity, steps should be taken to keep the bowels open. This may be accomplished with the use of natural aids. (Refer to chapter on bowel complaints.)

As a dietary supplement, one tablespoonful of lecithin granules obtained from soybeans may be taken twice daily. (Lecithin reputedly has a beneficial effect on the liver and gallbladder.) The granules may be sprinkled over food or added to fluids such as soups, coffee, or juices.

The amount of lecithin granules cited rarely if ever disagrees, but there are exceptions, and a few people find it too rich. In such cases the amount is simply reduced or may be completely cut out.

Case Histories

• "The fluid extract of an herb called fringe tree is one of the best remedies for bilious sick headache. I know, because it brought such great relief from the vicious attacks of migraine my poor mother suffered from. We learned of the remedy from a friend who heard about it from a Chinese herbalist." G.C.

• Mrs. Marjorie L. has written an account of her experiences with homeopathic Chionanthus (fringe tree). She says:

"For over ten years I suffered frequent attacks of the most dreadful migraine headaches, accompanied by dizzy spells, nausea, vomiting of bile, and an overwhelming sense of depression. At first these bouts were occasional, but as the years passed they came more often and lasted longer, until I had only about four or five days out of a month that I was not suffering from migraine. Although it is said that migraine is never fatal I sometimes found myself wishing that it was. The many doctors I visited were unable to help me.

"Then one day I happened to read an article by a woman who claimed she had cured herself of migraine headaches with the use of homeopathic Chionanthus 6X. I confess that I really didn't think the remedy would help me, but I was desperate so I thought I'd give it a try. I sent for the preparation from a homeopathic pharmacy and took the tiny Chionanthus pellets according to the directions on the bottle.

"As the weeks passed I was amazed to find that the vicious migraine attacks were growing less violent and occurring far less often. And for the first time in years my dreadfully pale cheeks had some color and my eyes lost their dark sunken look. I could hardly believe the miracle that was happening!

"I have taken the Chionanthus remedy faithfully for several months now, and what a marvelous new lease on life it has given me! I can't praise it enough. I am entirely free of migraine headache and all its old horrors. No longer am I forced to spend all my days in bed. Instead I am now leading an active and happy existence once more. I often pause in my busy rounds these days to thank God for giving us the precious little fringe tree!"

BARLEY WATER
AS AN AID IN JAUNDICE

Dr. Vogel of Switzerland states that the use of barley water has been found to be an effective remedy for conditions of jaundice. He writes:[3]

> This is confirmed by the report from a woman who contracted a severe jaundice and cured herself by this means alone: She boiled a cup of barley grains in 6 to 8 pints of water till they were soft, and drank the water during the day. The urine became quite clear and the jaundice disappeared. This sounds almost too simple to be true, but if it really helps, why should we not try it? I myself was very pleased with her story but not too surprised, because I knew of similar results being achieved in the tropics in the case of liver troubles and jaundice by the same means. Internal heat and fever respond very well to barley water too, for it imparts decided benefit to the kidneys as well as to the liver. However unassuming a medicine it may be, we can profitably use it in conjunction with other natural remedies and thus make still more certain of success. At the same time, it is an invaluable standby if no other remedies can be procured. Depending upon circumstances and the recuperative power of one's constitution it may very well be that barley water, physical measures, and the appropriate diet will be sufficient in themselves to bring about an entirely satisfactory cure.

LIVER DIET

Dr. Vogel suggests the following diet:[4]

> If sweet and fatty dishes do not agree with you, you may assume that your liver is not working as it should and that you must be careful. Radishes are an excellent remedy for the liver but you must take them only in small quantities. A teaspoonful of raw radish juice per day is the largest dose permissible. Raw carrot juice is almost a specific for the liver and, obtained in the same way as the juice of potatoes, will, if taken for a couple of days to the exclusion of everything else, work wonders. Needless to say, the carrots can be taken finely grated if the juice-extracting business proves to cumbersome. Bitter salads consisting of dandelion leaves, chicory and other bitter herbs (most of these act beneficially on the liver) will add to the favorable effect of the carrot

---

[3]*Ibid*, p. 103.

[4]*The Nature Doctor*, Bioforce-Verlag, Teufen (AR), Switzerland, 1959.

diet. Sweet and fat foods, even fruit juices, should be banned from the diet while you undergo this treatment; before long the liver will work again without giving you trouble, and vomiting of bile, which may have occurred, will have stopped, too.

The following will help you to avoid mistakes while you try to pacify your liver by means of diet:

Mornings: 1 glass carrot juice, a slice of toast or crisp bread with very little butter or yeast extract, some wheat germ.

Midday: Vegetable soup, brown rice or potatoes steamed in their jackets, chicory and raw carrot salad (or any other fresh salad such as endive, i.e., bitter ones to be preferred). Steamed vegetables may also be added to the lunch table. Fried and sweet dessert dishes must be avoided.

Variety in the lunch menu can be offered, too:

1st day: Brown rice, fennel-root, mixed salad.

2nd day: Potatoes steamed in their skins with a little cottage cheese, a little butter, and diverse salads.

3rd day: Vegetable soup, ryvita, wholemeal, or rye bread sandwiches prepared with butter, yeast extract, garlic, onions and slices of tomatoes; usual salads. A cereal coffee with a little milk but no sugar can be served afterwards.

Evening: Oat, barley, or unpolished rice soup with a few added vegetables; diverse salads seasoned with lemon juice, sour whey or sour milk (never with vinegar). For the sake of variety, sandwiches and salads with following cereal coffee may be served for supper.

Fruit is taboo while the liver is out of order.

SUMMARY

1. The liver is a remarkable chemical factory which detoxifies poisons that would otherwise pass into our blood.

2. The gallbladder stores and concentrates bile. If the flow of bile is sluggish, thick, or congested, a host of problems can occur.

3. Some authorities maintain that liver trouble is one of the most common among the many causes of migraine headache, due to a back-up of bile into the bloodstream.

4. Gallstones can be formed from different substances, but the cholesterol type is regarded as the easiest to dissolve.

5. Olive oil has been known to remove (not dissolve) gallstones, but should not be used if an X-ray reveals a large stone as it may become lodged in the bile duct.

6. A special diet should be used in addition to any of the remedies for gallbladder or liver ailments.

CHAPTER 3

Herbs for Coping with Stomach Ailments

Countless people the world over suffer from digestive disturbances which result in symptoms such as nausea, gas bloat, belching, stomach pains, coated tongue, a distressed feeling in the stomach after eating, sour eructions, foul breath, a bad taste in the mouth, and sometimes difficult breathing and palpitations.

Following is a list of herbs which may be used as aids to tone up the stomach, or as remedies for digestive ailments.

FENNEL

Botanical Name: *Foeniculum vulgare*
Common Name: Sweet Fennel

Fennel, "the friend of the stomach," has been used since earliest times as a culinary herb and medicine. It reputedly imparts a soothing effect to mucous membranes, and effectively helps people troubled with excessive belching and flatulence. In many lands it is used in cookery as an aid in the digestion of fish, beans, cabbage, peas, and cheese. Fennel seed steeped in olive oil makes a tasty dressing which greatly assists the digestibility of raw vegetable salads and also helps to prevent the formation of gas.

In Grandma's time people used a light, bland diet, and

drank four or five cups of pleasant-tasting fennel seed tea a day for several days following an upset stomach or stomach distress. Fennel tea is made by placing two teaspoonfuls of the seed in a half-cup of boiling water. Boil one minute, cover the vessel to retain the aromatic oil, strain and allow to become just warm.

GOLDEN SEAL

Botanical Name: *Hydrastis canadensis*
Common Names: Yellow Root, Indian Plant, Yellow Puccoon, Eye Balm

Indian tribes of North America relied almost entirely on the plant kingdom for their medicinal needs. One of the favorite herbs of the Cherokees was golden seal. This small perennial plant with a thick, fleshy yellow rhizome, produces a solitary rose-colored or whitish flower. The fruit somewhat resembles the raspberry, but is not edible.

This plant grows in moist, rich woodlands in various parts of the United States, but more abundantly in the northeastern sections. The name "golden seal" was given to the herb because of the seal-like scars on the golden-yellow root. In botany it is known as *Hydrastis canadensis*.

The first medical reference to golden seal appeared in Barton's *Collection for a Vegetable Materia Medica* (1798), in which he credits the Cherokee Indians with the introduction of the plant to the settlers. Hand (*House Surgeon*, 1820) also referred to the plant and stated that it "may be given in form of powder or strong tea made by boiling, in indigestion, the secondary stages of low fevers and in all cases of weakness in general."

Rafinesque, in his *Medical Flora of the United States* (1828), defined the yellow alkaloid of golden seal as a "peculiar principle hydrastine of a yellow color." He devoted considerable attention to the plant, and stated: "Internally it is used as a bitter tonic in infusion or tincture in disorders of the stomach, liver, etc."

Golden Seal in the 20th Century

Golden seal is classified as restorative, bitter, tonic, antiseptic, and alterative. The tea is pleasantly bitter and somewhat pungent to the taste.

William Fox, M.D., employed golden seal as a stimulating tonic which "has a powerful action upon the mucous membranes, which renders it useful in cases of gastric debility and indigestion."

Drs. Wood and Ruddock cited golden seal as a remedy in various disorders. They especially valued it in the treatment of "some forms of dyspepsia" and recommended the decoction in the dose of "one tablespoonful three times a day; of the tincture, one to two teaspoonfuls three times a day."

In a modern British volume on botanical drugs, golden seal is cited as a valuable remedy in disordered states of the digestive system. "As a general bitter tonic it is applicable to debilitated conditions of the mucous tissues. As a remedy for various gastric disorders it takes a leading place, acting very beneficially in acute inflammatory conditions. It will be found of value in all cases of dyspepsia, biliousness, and debility of the system.

Mattson suggests one teaspoon of golden seal powder steeped in one-half cup of hot water. It may be sweetened to make it more palatable. Putting the powder in empty capsules which are then swallowed with a little water is another popular method of using golden seal.

Frank Roberts, a medical herbalist of England, refers to golden seal as a remedy "par excellence" for stomach troubles. He writes:

> Under its influence, the gastric and intestinal secretions are increased or restored to normal both in quantity and quality.
>
> Peristalsis (or wave-like pushing-onwards activity of the intestines) is gently stimulated so that costiveness is relieved in a gentle and natural manner. In fact, golden seal is the most natural and gentle of stimulants to all the digestive functions. It influences the mucous surfaces and is therefore clearly indicated in the treatment of gastric and duodenal ulcers, catarrh of the stomach, acute and chronic gastritis and other irritable conditions of the stomach and intestines, including colitis and enteritis.
>
> If the stomach is inactive or lacking in tone or "nervous" in any way, this remedy will be found second to none, improving the appetite, normalizing the digestive juices, and favorably influencing all digestive processes. In all simple digestive problems, e.g., indigestion or dyspepsia, it will give rapid relief and cure.

ROSEMARY

Botanical Name: *Rosmarinus officinalis*
Common Names: Rosmarin, Romero

Rosemary belongs to the mint family. The botanical name

is from the Latin *ros* (dew) and *marinus* (of the sea), as the plant grows luxuriously near the seashore. There are several varieties under cultivation in gardens, *Rosmarinus officinalis* being the more common and popular species.

In former times the Greeks and Romans burned the fragrant plant as incense during their religious rites, and crowned their guests of honor with garlands made from the leaves. Because the herb was used as a crowning wreath it was often called *Rosmarinus coronaria*.

Rosemary was grown in the gardens of the early monks for use as a medicinal agent. The young leaves, tops, and flowers were prepared as a tea for treating stomach disorders, nervousness, and other ailments.

Rosemary—a Valuable Herb

Rosemary is classified as carminative, aromatic, tonic, astringent, and diaphoretic. Until recent years, the leaves of this herb were mixed with juniper twigs and burned regularly in French hospital wards to purify the air and to check the spread of infection. In various parts of the world, common rosemary is used mainly as a stomachic and nervine. A medicinal water distilled from the plant is highly esteemed in Hungary for nervous ailments and digestive disorders.

Fr. Kneipp of Germany referred to rosemary as an excellent stomachic. "Prepared as a tea it [rosemary] cleanses the stomach of phlegm, gives a good appetite and good digestion. Whoever likes to see the medicine glass, this comforter in illness shining on his table, let him fill it with rosemary tea, and take from two to four tablespoonfuls morning and evening. The stomach will soon become sensible, that is, it will not stick fast much longer in phlegm."

Rosemary tea is prepared in the same manner as ordinary tea.

OKRA

Botanical Name: *Hibiscus esculentis*
Common Name: Okra

Because of its mucilaginous and bland nature, okra is highly valued as a demulcent food. Demulcents are prized for their protective coating-like properties and are used internally to relieve irritation of membranes.

Powdered okra may be taken with water, or with bland foods such as broths or milk.

As a Remedy for Stomach Ulcers

The following was reported by Dr. Herman N. Bundesen:

"It was observed by a certain doctor that a patient who had mucous colitis, a disorder in which there are alternating attacks of constipation and diarrhea, was improved by using a large amount of ... okra.... This observation led Dr. J. Meyer of Chicago and his co-workers to make a study of okra.

"They used a dry powdered okra in treating ulcer of the stomach and first part of the intestine. This okra is a light yellow-green color and has a fairly pleasant taste. When mixed with water, the powder becomes thick. However, the powdered okra was given to the patients in the form of tablets or capsule.

"Seventeen persons with ulcer of the stomach or the first part of the intestines were given powdered okra as the only form of treatment for their condition. The diagnosis was made in each case by means of X-ray. All of the patients were having symptoms of ulcer of the stomach or first part of the intestine at the time the treatment was started.

"Of the seventeen patients who were treated, fourteen obtained immediate relief from their symptoms with the powdered okra treatment. One individual had no relief for three days after starting the okra treatment, but on the fifth day his symptoms did disappear.

"Evidently then this powdered okra does give quick relief from the symptoms of ulcers. ..."

In reference to the study mentioned above, another American physician, Dr. Evans, had this to say: "Our old friend okra seems on the point of assuming new duties and responsibilities. The new job it is taking on is that of relieving the discomfort of ulcer of the stomach. It threatens to push bicarbonate of soda and mucin out of their chief employment as a medicine.

"A few years ago it occurred to some physicians that if 'gooey' stuff from animal sources was of service in treating the pain and discomfort of stomach ulcer, similar material of vegetable origin might have the same effect and yet be more pleasant to take. ... Then it was recalled that okra ... because of some mucilaginous content, might be worthy of trial.

"Different groups have been using it for several months. Drs. J. Meyer, E. E. Seidmon, and H. Necheles published a report of seventeen cases. The results obtained were quite as good as those given by any other treatment.

"As a rule, the users like to chew the okra tablets. The treatment was popular both on its own account and also because it was a means of escape from unpleasant 'goos'. It was found taking okra powder not only eased the discomfort but also caused the stomach to empty more promptly. . . ."

RED CENTAURY

Botanical Name: *Erythraea centaurium*
Common Names: Centaury, Filwort

Red century is native to Europe and North Africa. Its botanical name, *Erythrea*, is drived from the Greek *erythros* (red) from the color of the flowers. It was formerly named Chironia, from Chiron of Greek mythology who was skilled in using medicinal herbs.

Modern Usage

The action of red centaury is classified by medical herbalists as aromatic, tonic, bitter, and stomachic. It is used extensively for conditions of dyspepsia, heart burn, and poor appetite. The herb is prepared as a tea, one ounce to one pint of water. One small cupful is taken one-half hour before meals.

OLIVE

Botanical Name: *Olea europaea*
Common Name: Olive

Olive oil is easily digested and imparts a generally soothing and healing influence to the digestive tract.

In a medical health publication, *Hamdard Digest* (India), Dr. J. Dewitt Fox writes that he treats his ulcer patients with olive oil. He relates an incident of a young friend of his, a Mexican doctor, who took him to dinner at a restaurant in Mexico. Dr. Fox was astonished at the amount of hot sauce his friend consumed without the slightest indication of stomach distress. When questioned about this, his friend replied that he takes a little olive oil first, as it protects his stomach.

Dr. Fox suggests substituting olive oil for the cream generally advised as part of the ulcer diet. "Two tablespoons of olive oil with, or followed by, six ounces of milk will do the same or even a better job of healing than the cream. It will also reduce stomach acids, and because the oil is unsaturated will not raise the blood cholesterol."

Some medical men speculate that olive oil may contain vitamin U, a substance which is believed to have a healing influence on ulcers.

GENTIAN

Botanical Name: *Gentiana lutea*
Common Name: Gentian

There are many varieties of gentian, although not all are employed as medicines. One species which is widely used as a therapeutic agent is the yellow-flowered gentian, known botanically as *Gentiana lutea*. It grows in central and southern Europe, especially on the Pyrenees and the Alps. The root, which is imported, has an intensely bitter taste and is the only part of the plant that contains medicinal properties.

Gentian was named after Gentius, king of Illyria, who was also a botany student. He is reputed to have been the first to discover the remedial value of the plant which bears his name. Over a dozen remedies were credited to it at that time. It was used for debility, fatigue, derangement of the stomach, and liver disorders. A wine in which the root had been steeped was considered excellent for chills due to exposure. Many of the complex preparations handed down from the Arabians and Greeks contain gentian as one of their ingredients.

Gentian Bitters

Bitters is the popular name for a liquor in which a bitter herb, root, or leaf has been macerated. They are used as tonics or stimulants to increase the appetite and to improve digestion.

The custom of employing bitters as a stomach tonic is age-old. The ancient Romans, notorious for their food orgies, were convinced that bitters were important for digestion. Dr. J. Paris of the Royal College of Physicians said, "It may be laid down as a truth, that bitters stimulate the stomach." The American Indians also appreciated the natural bitter of herbs, vegetables, and fruits.

Today, gentian enters largely into the composition of many

different formulas for bitters and is very popular in the mountain-
ous regions of Germany and Switzerland, where it is known as
Enzien.

Gentian Bitters as a Remedy

Bitters can be made either with a single botanical or as a
special combination of herbs, depending upon the flower and
action desired. Taken before meals, they stimulate the appetite
and impart a beneficial influence to the stomach. They are especially valued by people inclined to a sedentary mode of life.

Father Kneipp, of European fame, strongly advocated the
use of gentian bitters. He wrote:

> Before all, I advise you to prepare extract of gentian. The gen-
> tian roots are for this purpose well dried, cut small, and then put
> into bottles with brandy or spirit. [Steep for one week, then strain.]
>
> This extract is one of the best stomachics. Put six to eight
> tablespoonfuls of water into a glass, and pour in 20 to 30 drops
> of extract; take this mixture daily for some time. The good diges-
> tion will soon be indicated by a no less good appetite. If the food
> is felt to be heavy in the stomach, and is troublesome, a little
> cordial made with a teaspoonful of extract in half a glass of water,
> will soon stop the disorder.
>
> Gentian is likewise very good for cramp in the stomach. When
> after a long journey during which for days together eating fares
> badly and drinking still worse, people arrive at their destination
> dead tired and almost ill, a tiny bottle of gentian tincture taken
> by drops on sugar, will render excellent services.
>
> Nausea and attacks of faintness are removed by taking a tea-
> spoonful of tincture in water; it warms, enlivens, and brings body
> and mind to peace again.

Dr. Swinburne Clymer gives his medical opinion of gentian
bitters as follows:

> An activated, safe stomach bitters of great value. Gentian is
> always indicated when the activity of the digestive organism is
> enfeebled, and where there is nausea and faint feeling due to
> indigestion. It is best combined with other agents such as *Hydras-
> tis* (golden seal). In slow digestion it is always indicated as it will
> speed up the digestive powers and aid digestion of food. It will
> irritate in large doses, but in small doses reduces irritation of the
> mucous membranes. In mental weariness, and depression over
> the solar plexus, it is the first agent indicated. Dose, of the tincture,
> 3 to 20 drops [in a small glass of water].

NOTE: Prepared herbal tinctures may be obtained from various herb firms.

SLIPPERY ELM

Botanical Name: *Ulmus fulva*
Common Names: Red Elm, American Elm, Indian Elm

Slippery elm is a small tree which grows in various parts of North America. The inner bark was an important food and medicine of the American Indians and pioneers. As a healing agent it was prepared and used as a tea so that its soothing properties could reach deep-seated delicate membranes of the throat as well as irritations of the stomach and intestines. The bark was also employed in the form of a poultice for wounds, burns, etc.

Modern Usage of Slippery Elm

Slippery elm has wonderful and strengthening qualities. It is considered one of nature's finest demulcents and is used for its ability to absorb noxious gases in the body and to neutralize stomach acidity. It is also recognized for its soothing action in minor peptic irritations of the stomach and intestines. When the powdered bark is prepared as a gruel it forms a wholesome and nutritious food. It is especially valuable for the elderly and those with touchy digestion or recuperating from illnesses.

Because of its mucilagnous nature, slippery elm insures easy passage during the process of assimilation and elimination. Its action is so gentle that it can be retained by delicate stomachs when other foods are rejected. It also acts as a buffer against irritation and inflammation of the mucous membranes.

As an herbal tea, slippery elm bark is generally prepared by mixing two teaspoonfuls of the powdered bark in a half-cup of cold water. This is placed in a container and shaken thoroughly. One pint of boiling water is then added and the mixture well stirred. Herbalists prescribe that the tea be taken three times daily.

The gruel is made by heating a half-pint of milk and sprinkling one-half to one teaspoonful of powdered slippery elm bark into the liquid. This is beaten thoroughly with an egg beater or electric mixer, then brought to a boil and stirred until it thickens. It may be sweetened with honey. Some people prefer to beat up an egg with one teaspoonful of the powdered bark. Boiling milk is then poured over the mixture which is stirred well and sweetened to taste.

ANISE

Botanical Name: *Pimpinella anisum*
Common Name: Anise

Anise is a dainty, white-flowered annual about 18 inches high; when cultivated the plant attains considerably larger size. It is native to Egypt, Greece, and Asia Minor.

Anise is one of the oldest plants known and has been employed as a spice and domestic medicine. It was used by the ancient Egyptians, and later cultivated in the imperial German farms of Charlemagne.

Anise has a long-standing reputation as a carminative, stomachic, and flavoring agent. Several centuries ago the Romans and Greeks used anise in relishes, sauces, and wines. The seeds were chewed as a breath sweetener and to stimulate the appetite. The Romans served a wedding cake strongly flavored with anise seeds to help prevent indigestion caused by overeating at the marriage banquet. From this ancient practice came the tradition of baking special cakes for weddings.

In Europe and other lands, anise tea is considered a good domestic remedy for preventing gas and fermentation in the stomach and bowels. The tea is prepared by placing a teaspoonful of the seeds in a cup and adding hot water. The cup is covered with a saucer, and the brew allowed to steep for a few minutes, then strained. The tea is taken in doses of a teaspoonful to a tablespoonful (repeated often).

PAPAYA

Botanical Name: *Carica payaya*
Common Name: Papaya

The papaya is a melon-like tropical fruit which is produced in clusters by the *Carica papaya* tree. In certain regions of the tropics it is regarded by the natives as a mystical plant because in some ways it appears to possess human attributes, producing male and female flowers on separate plants, while the fruit, like the human embryo, develops in about nine months.

Papaya Known to Early Explorers

Papaya is frequently cited in the writings of the early explorers. Columbus was impressed by the fact that the natives of the Caribbean could eat exceptionally heavy meals of fish and meat without any apparent discomfort if the meal was followed by a dessert of papaya. Magellan regarded it as a valuable article of the diet. According to Ponce de Leon, natives called it Vanti, a word that meant "keep well."

The Medicine Tree

Papaya is often referred to as the Medicine Tree, as almost every part of the tree is believed to contain medicinal properties. The unripe fruit as well as other parts of the plant contain a powerful protein-digesting enzyme called papain which greatly resembles pepsin in its digestive action.

Protein foods decompose more rapidly than other foods, and the longer they are retained in the intestinal tract the more likely they are to cause a toxic condition. This can result in gas, foul mouth taste, foul breath, constipation, sour stomach, stomach distresses, and heartburn.

The natural papain enzyme is extracted from the unripe papaya melon, made into tablets, and sold as an aid to protein digestion. They are especially effective upon meat, and increase its utilization by making it more assimilable. They also improve the utilization of fats, starches, and carbohydrates as well as the protein contained in plant foods such as beans, peas, nuts, and lentils. The tablets also help in the digestion of meals cooked in grease or fats.

Interesting Cases

One woman wrote, "I am so happy since I found out about papaya tablets. I was always filled with gas—even water caused gas. This has disappeared like magic since taking them." In another case there was a man plagued with dyspepsia, much to the concern of his wife. She complained, "He could clutch his middle and issue a series of little moans like owls wailing among the ruins of some buried city. Papain killed all the owls and now he's fairly hooting for his fish and chips."

ACACIA

Botanical Name: *Acacia vera*
Common Names: Gum Arabic, Gum Acacia

The acacia is a small tree or shrub, which sometimes attains considerable height. The gum flows from the bark in the form of thick liquid which quickly concretes into tears.

Gum arabic is classified as nutritive and demulcent. Its nutritional properties were recognized by desert tribesmen who sometimes lived on it entirely during the gum harvest.

Modern Usage

Pulverized gum arabic is considered a food remedy of great value in cases where the membranes of the digestive and assimilative system are involved. It possesses soothing and healing properties.

Dr. Eric Powell of England recommends the following:

"For curative purposes dissolve a teaspoonful of acacia in a cup of hot water; add a pinch of cinnamon and a little honey if desired. Take a cupful in sips a few minutes before meals three times daily. In circumstances where digestion is very poor and there is much inflammation of the vital organs of digestion and elimination, take a cupful four times daily and go without food for two or three days. Taken during tasting, this preparation will promote rapid healing of the inflamed surfaces and at the same time provide all the nourishment necessary for the time being. This method of taking acacia has resulted in the cure of gastritis, duodenal ulceration, ulceration of the intestines, and inflammation of the kidneys and bladder. In severe cases the remedy taken while fasting should be adopted for two days out of every seven while the trouble lasts, and taken before meals on all other days.

"The gum is perfectly harmless to all ages, and the quantity stated as a dose may be exceeded if necessary without any adverse effects."

HONEY

The use of honey as a food and natural medicine is age-old. It is mentioned in the Bible, the Koran, and the sacred texts of China, Egypt, and India as an excellent remedy and wholesome component of the diet. King Solomon, reknown for his wisdom, advised, "My son, eat thou honey, for it is good." (Pro. 24:13.) Mohammed proclaimed, "Honey is a remedy for all diseases."

Honey was also in great demand as a remedial agent in Greece, and in the Roman Empire. Its main employment was as a remedy for gastric and intestinal disorders, respiratory troubles, kidney ailments, and as a gentle laxative. It was also extensively used for inflammation of the eyes and eyelids.

The early herbalists also employed honey for similar ailments.

Modern Remedial Uses of Honey

Honey is a popular home remedy in many European countries and among Asiatic races. It is employed for a variety of complaints but is considered of especially great value for digestive disorders. Its flavor stimulates the appetite and aids digestion. For dyspeptics, convalescents, and the aged, honey is regarded as a highly effective tonic and reconstructive.

Several eminent European gastroenterologists recommend the use of honey for hyperacidity, gastric catarrh, and peptic ulcers. For example, Dr. Schacht of Wiesbaden claims to have successfully treated many cases with honey.

Constituents in Honey

Honey contains protein, minerals, fatty acids, vitamins B, C, and K, riboflavin, thiamin, niacin, and other life-giving substances. It is non-irritating to the lining of the digestive tract. Its fatty acid content stimulates peristalsis. Honey does not ferment in the stomach. It is rapidly and easily assimilated as it has been predigested by the bees, making it unnecessary for the human gastro-intestinal tract to do this additional work.

Some Interesting Case Histories

• A woman, age 30, took several teaspoonfuls of buckwheat honey every day during the hay fever season to prevent hay fever. When the season ended, she was astonished to find that a long-standing ulcer condition had vanished.

• A salesman in his early forties suffered periodic bouts of ulcer pains. Buckwheat honey cleared up the ulcer condition and he reports that he still takes the honey daily as a preventative against any recurrence of the trouble.

SUMMARY

1. Digestive disturbances can result in symptoms such as gas bloat, belching, nausea, sour eructions, stomach pains, foul breath, a bad taste in the mouth, stomach distress after eating, and sometimes difficult breathing and palpitations.

2. Many botanicals provided by nature have been effectively used the world over to tone up the stomach, and to relieve certain digestive ailments.

3. Selected herbs have successfully coped with some cases of peptic ulcers.

4. Herb bitters are used as tonics or stimulants to promote a lagging appetite, and to improve digestion.

CHAPTER 4

Herb Remedies for Respiratory Disorders

After his travels through the interior of Africa, the early French explorer Francois Levaillant gave an account of the plant medicine used by the natives. He reported that they administered an herbal remedy that cured him of quinsy* after he had considered his case hopeless.

Due to severe swelling of the throat and tongue, Levaillant could communicate only by signs. For almost a week he had despaired of his life, and his breathing had become so dangerously impeded that he expected to suffocate at any moment. He was visited during the evening by a party of natives who took an interest in his condition and pledged themselves to help him.

A hot herbal poultice was bound to his throat, and additional covering placed over this to retain the heat as long as possible. As soon as the poultice began to cool it was immediately replaced with another, and the hot poulticing was continued throughout the night. In addition a gargle was prepared from the same plant and used repeatedly. By daybreak the inflammation and swelling had greatly subsided and Levaillant could breathe more freely. Both methods of using the herbal

---

*Quinsy is a severe infection of the tonsil associated with the formation of an abscess alongside the tonsil.

remedy were continued, and by the third day he considered himself completely well.

Determined to examine the plant which had restored his health, he was astonished to find that "nothing in the country was more common; it grew all around the camp and was to be met with in every direction." Levaillent says that the herb was a species of ordinary sage, about two feet in height, with a balsamic taste and fragrant odor.

Let us consider this remarkable herb and some of the many others that have been used in different parts of the world for treating respiratory ailments.

SAGE

Botanical Name: *Salvia officinalis*
Common Name: Common Sage

This is a perennial plant reaching about two feet in height, bearing blue flowers variegated with purple and white. The leaves are a grayish-green color sometimes tinged with purple or red. For centuries sage has been cultivated for culinary and medicinal purposes in England, France, and Germany. The Latin name for sage (*Salvia officinalis*) is a derivation of *salvere*, "to be saved," in reference to the therapeutic properties of the plant.

What Sage Contains

In pharmaceutical writings, sage is listed among the natural antiseptics. It contains a volatile oil, tannin, resin, and a bitter principle. The oil is composed of pinene, camphor, salvene, and cineol. Brieskorn and Schlumprecht discovered ursolic acid in sage leaves. Sage oil also contains bactericidal properties.

Medicinal Uses

Medical herbalists employ sage in conditions of tonsillitis, quinsy, and ulceration of the mouth and throat. For these purposes a preparation is made by pouring a half-pint of hot malt vinegar over one ounce of sage leaves. A half-pint of water is added. This is taken frequently in wineglassful doses and is also used as a gargle.

Another formula which may be used as a gargle for tonsillitis consists of pouring one quart of boiling water over two ounces of sage. This is allowed to stand for two hours, then strained, and a small bit of pulverized alum added.

One woman who tried the sage-alum gargle wrote: "My oldest boy woke up with tonsillitis one morning, so I prepared a tea of sage and alum and had him gargle with it several times a day. The next day he was rid of the tonsillitis, where other times he would suffer for weeks and could not eat or sleep."

In various European countries sage preparations such as extracts, tinctures, infusions, and so forth, are used for easing bronchitis and inflammation of the throat, and as gargles and mouth washes.

The following item appeared in a British health publication:[1]

Garden sage, a simple aromatic astringent, has recently undergone a series of tests. As most herbalists know, it makes an excellent gargle for sore throats and needs no introduction into the treatment of aphthous ulcers. It has been used with success for pharyngitis, Vincent's angina, stomatitis, and glossitis [inflammation of the tongue].

A bactericide and fungicide (antiseptic) of subtle and penetrating power, it scores a definite victory over penicillin-resistant substances and common oral pathogens. It is singularly helpful in oral thrush [a fungus disease of the mouth].

Dr. Bartram of England presents the following:[2]

For laryngitis and pharyngitis an infusion of sage can be made by placing a handful of the leaves in a pint of boiling water, and covering until cool to prevent the escape of volatile properties. Excellent for catarrh. One wineglassful can be taken, after straining, between meals, three times daily. Of special value for buccal ulcers [sores of mouth or tongue] and tonsillitis. Tonsils should not be removed unless really necessary. They are the centre of lymphatic protection of the throat. They are one of nature's gardeners against infectious disease. Seven of the vocal muscles originate in the sheath of the tonsils. When extirpated, the undue relaxation of these muscles impairs pharyngeal control and vocal resonance.

ONION

Botanical Name: *Allium cepa*
Common Name: Common Onion

The onion belongs to the same botanical family as garlic, and is one of the oldest vegetables known to man. It has been

---

[1] *Health from Herbs*, July–August 1967.
[2] *Grace Magazine*, autumn 1960.

cultivated since the remote past, as references in Hebrew and Sanskrit literature indicate. Because of the sheaths which envelop the bulb, the Egyptians regarded it as a symbol of the universe.

Constituents and Uses

Raw onions contain an acrid volatile oil, phosphorus, calcium, magnesium, sulphur, sodium, potassium, iron, starch, acetic and phosphoric acids with phosphate and citrate of lime. They also contain vitamins A, B, C, and traces of iodine, zinc and silicon.

The onion has been used from past to present as a remedy for coughs, colds, and other respiratory ailments. In many European countries, hot onion poultices applied to the chest are considered helpful for bronchitis. In India onions are used as a home remedy for colds and coughs by slicing the fresh bulb and suspending the slices near the patient.

A syrup made from the juice of an onion mixed with honey was regarded by Dr. Fernie as an excellent remedy for phlegm when the lungs are congested and breathing is difficult. Drs. Wood and Ruddock presented the following information:

Croup. The French remedy for croup is onions. Cut them into thin slices, sprinkling each slice with a layer of sugar. This will soon yield a syrup of which a teaspoonful should be taken about every fifteen minutes until relief is obtained.

Bronchitis.

Simple syrup—three tablespoonfuls
Onion juice—two tablespoonfuls
Dose: One teaspoonful before meals

Or, slice the onions, sprinkle sugar over them; let stand an hour or two, then mash and press out the juice. Dose: one teaspoonful three times a day and before retiring at night. In severe cases, every three hours.

Onions also have an excellent reputation for curing the type of cold characterized by watering of the eyes and a watery constant discharge from the nose. For example, Dr. Vogel of Switzerland writes:[3]

Colds. A "streaming" cold, the symptoms of which are bland lachrymation and excoriating nasal discharge, will always be

---

[3]*The Nature Doctor,* Bioforce-Verlag, Teufen (AR), Switzerland, 1959.

helped by onions. Their Latin name is *Allium cepa*, and as such they are well known to every homeopath. What you have to do to get rid of that type of cold is simple enough; just cut a slice from a fresh raw onion and immerse it quickly in a glass of hot water. Do not let it remain in the water for longer than a second or so. Take little sips of this water throughout the day. If the above-mentioned symptoms correspond with your own, your cold will soon leave you. In addition, you may cut an onion in half and put it on your bedside table so you can breathe in the smell during your sleep.

Onion Therapy Used by a French Doctor

A French army physician used fresh onion juice to treat grippe patients by giving them 200 cubic centimeters of the juice in hot tea, divided into three doses, each day. This treatment was administered as soon as the disease had first started. In two days the fever was gone. There were no fatalities among the patients who were given the onion treatment.

Hay Fever and Colds.

Dr. Bartram of England recommends the homeopathic form of onion for hay fever: "four pilules, 6X potency, three times daily, between meals until relief is felt."[4]

He also recommends the same form for the following: "Streaming cold. Profuse watery discharge from nose and eyes. eyes inflamed. Often painful tearing cough. Easier in the open air or in a cold room. Four pilules, 6X potency, every two hours."[5]

Another English herbalist claims the following remedy works like magic for conditions of asthma. He advises placing a few thin slices of raw onions on a plate. Honey is then spread on each slice, and the preparation is covered with an inverted plate, allowing it to stand overnight. A teaspoonful of the resulting syrup is taken four times a day.

PLEURISY ROOT

Botanical Name: *Asclepias tuberosa*
Common Names: Butterfly Weed, Wind Root, Tuber Root

Pleurisy root is a perennial plant, bearing deep yellow and

---

[4]*Grace*, Autumn 1963.
[5]*Ibid*, winter 1960.

orange flowers. The rootstock, which is spindle-shaped with a knotty crown, is the part of the plant used in herbal medicine.

Remedial Use of Pleurisy Root

Herbalists classify the medicinal action of pleurisy root as diaphoretic, antispasmodic, expectorant, carminative, and tonic. It reputedly has a specific action on the lungs, subdues inflammation, loosens phlegm, and exerts a mild tonic effect on the system. As its name implies, it is considered of great value as a remedy for conditions of pleurisy, relieving the pain and the difficulty of breathing.

The tea is prepared by stirring one teaspoon of pleurisy root powder in one cup of boiling water. One cupful is taken warm every hour to induce free perspiration and promote expectoration, then the dosage is reduced to one cupful three times a day.

If the fluid extract is used, one-half to one teaspoonful is taken in a small glass of warm water three or four times daily.

Accessory Treatment

As an accessory treatment, hot herbal fomentations are applied to the painful side. Two ounces of pleurisy root are boiled in one quart of water for 10 minutes, then strained. A flannel is wrung out in the decoction and placed on the affected area as hot as can be comfortably borne. The flannel is covered with a dry towel to retain the heat. As soon as the fomentation begins to cool it is renewed, and the hot fomentations are continued until relief is obtained.

VIOLET

Botanical Name: *Viola odorata*
Common Name: Sweet-scented Violet

The Greeks and Romans used violets in food and drink. The Chinese use a species of violet as a pot herb. As early as the 14th century, violet jelly and violet fritters were served as dishes in England.

Medicinal Uses

Herbalists recommend a tea prepared from violets for chronic coughs and catarrh. It is also considered an excellent gargle for sore throats. The tea is made by placing a small handful of the dried leaves in a saucepan with two teacupfuls of cold water. This is brought to a boil and then immediately removed. When cold, the beverage is strained, and a half-teacupful is taken morning and evening after meals.

Fr. Kneipp, the famed German herbalist, wrote:

> When in the beginning of spring-time, the children get bad coughs in consequence of the frequent changes in the weather, the anxious mother boils a handful of green or dried violet leaves in half a pint of water, and gives the children two or three spoonfuls of such tea every two or three hours. Adults are cured of whooping-cough by taking a cup of this tea three times a day.

> It likewise relieves the cough of consumptive people and assists in loosening the phlegm. It serves as a medicine and should be taken as such, i.e., three to five tablespoonfuls every two or three hours.

> For swollen throat this tea is a tested gargle; at the same time the throat-bandage* may be applied, dipped in the decoction instead of pure water.

> *NOTE: A piece of linen is immersed in the decoction, then wrung out and wound around the neck as an external application.

COMFREY

Botanical Name: *Symphytum officinalis*
Common Name: Knitbone, Common Comfrey

Comfrey has long been employed as a domestic remedy for asthma and other pulmonary complaints. It is also used for tonsillitis and quinsy sore throat.

For treating coughs, the root is considered more effective than the leaves, and is prepared by simmering one ounce of the roots in one quart of water for ten minutes. The decoction is allowed to stand until cold, then strained. It is reheated and one cupful taken twice daily.

If the leaves are used they are prepared as ordinary tea—one pint of boiling water poured over one ounce of the leaves. One cupful of the strained tea is taken three or four times a day.

Fresh comfrey leaves eaten daily have proved highly effective in some conditions of asthma, hay fever, and congestion. Mrs. Dorothy Johnson, B.H.Sc., of New Zealand, wrote: "A friend of mine, a cardiac and allergy asthmatic, nibbled absent-mindedly at the leaves while we discussed the virtues of comfrey in horse breeding. The next day he rang up in great excitement to tell me he had his first unbroken night's sleep in 30 years. For weeks he ate a little raw comfrey every day and slept through every night."

Mr. P., of British Columbia, kept records of a man who used pieces of comfrey root an inch long and about half an inch thick sliced like raw carrots in salad, and was happy to find these gave him relief from congestion in winter. Another very severe case reported that he eats eight to ten fresh comfrey leaves a day in sandwiches and salads and is no longer troubled by indigestion or congestion. He says he feels like a million dollars. One man who suffered from hay fever discovered that he could keep the condition completely under control by eating two or more six-inch fresh comfrey leaves daily throughout the hay fever season.

Mrs. L. N. writes: "Several years ago both my young daughter and I were suffering badly from bronchitis and asthma. My husband was very worried about us, and kept reading books about possible natural remedies, since orthodox medications were of little help. He came across many impressive reports about using the fresh leaves of a plant called comfrey, so he decided we should give it a try. Even though it was winter at the time, he was determined to grow the plants in our small hothouse, so he bought some root cuttings.

"The plants flourished under his care and he soon was able to trim off the tender tops which we ate every day as a salad or as a lightly boiled green vegetable. He also made a tea from the roots and we drank several cups daily. Within about a week we noticed an improvement in both the asthma and bronchitis symptoms, and could also sleep better at night.

"We continued to improve over a period of weeks until my daughter and I both felt completely cured. During the following spring we planted a dozen more plants outside in our regular garden where they grew into large lush plants which have given us a plentiful supply year after year. We also learned to dry the leaves in bunches and to sun-dry the roots which we also use as a tea. We have never stopped using this remarkable herb in one form or another, since we don't want a return of the hereditary asthma.

"Over the past years, a number of people with asthma have asked us for root cuttings and have grown and used the plant with excellent results. However, some of them said they found it more convenient to buy the dried roots from herb firms, for making the tea."

ELDER

Botanical Name: *Sambucus canadensis*
Common Names: Common Elder, Pipe Tree, Popgun Tree

The American elder, *Sambucus canadensis*, is a shrub reaching from six to twelve feet in height with small white flowers and purple-black or red berries. The common elder of Europe, known botanically as *Samucus nigra*, is larger, approaching the size of a tree.

Healthful Properties Contained in Elder

Elderberry tea has been employed for generations as a folk remedy for such conditions as colds, coughs, and influenza. Yet it was only in recent years that science discovered that elderberries contain *viburnic acid*, a substance which induces perspiration, and which is useful in cases of bronchitis and similar ailments. The berries also provide vitamins A, B, and C. A glucoside, *eldrin*, which is identical with rutin, is found in the flowers. In addition they contain a fragrant volatile oil and malates of potash and lime. Other constituents of the plant include fat, gum, starch, pectin, albumin, resin, grape sugar, and various alkaline and earthy salts.

Remedial Uses of Elder

As a domestic remedy, a tea made with one ounce of elder flowers to one pint of water is considered almost a specific for the alleviation of influenza. This simple infusion or tea is very popular in England where the sale of dried elder flowers has increased by 50 percent during the past several years. Elderberry wine taken hot with sugar or honey just before retiring at night is another well-known and popular remedy for colds.

A homeopathic tincture of elder is used to relieve asthma and croup. The dose is one to five drops in a small glass of water.

Elder-Peppermint Combination

The origin of this herbal combination for treating colds and influenza goes a long way back in folk medicine and has maintained its healing reputation right up to modern times. It reportedly promotes sweating, eliminates toxic matter through the skin, aids circulation, frees the respiratory organs, and increases the sufferer's vitality. It is claimed that many years ago, during an influenza epidemic, herbalists using the elder-peppermint combination never lost a case, while many patients under orthodox treatment died.

The tea is prepared by mixing together one-half ounce each of elder flowers and peppermint leaves. The mixture is placed in one pint of cold water and brought to a boil in a covered container. As soon as the water boils the container is removed and the tea allowed to stand for 20 minutes, then strained. The brew is reheated and taken hot, one teacupful every two hours, until symptoms are relieved.

Here is another recipe that is also considered very effective. A good handful each of elder flowers and peppermint leaves are well mixed and placed in a container. One and a half pints of boiling water are poured on, and the tea allowed to stand for 30 minutes. (The container should be covered to keep the steam from escaping.) The tea is then strained, reheated, and may be sweetened with honey. An adult may drink the whole brew while remaining in bed with a hot water bottle on the feet. The remedy is repeated the next day if necessary. Herbalists point out that since the tea produces sweating, it is important to remain in bed and keep warm.

YARROW

Botanical Name: *Achillea millefolium*
Common Names: Knight's Milfoil, Thousand Weed, Yarroway

Yarrow grows everywhere in fields, meadows, pastures, and roadsides. Its clusters of flowers are white or pale lilac, somewhat like miniature daisies in appearance. The botanical name of *Millefolium* is derived from the many segments of its leaves, hence its popular name of thousand weed.

Constituents and Uses

Yarrow yields a volatile oil containing *azuline* and *achilleine*, a glyco-alkaloid; also gum, tannin, resin, chlorides of calcium and potassium, and various salts.

Yarrow tea is used for different ailments but is especially regarded as a very good remedy for colds. It is sometimes called "Englishman's quinine" as it reputedly gets rid of a fever quickly and naturally. It is considered very effective where there are symptoms of chills and sensations of alternate cold and heat, and symptoms of constant nasal drip and catarrh.

The infusion is made by pouring one pint of boiling water over one ounce of the dried herb. The tea is steeped for five minutes, then strained and drunk warm in wineglassful doses. A pinch of cayenne pepper is added to each dose. The tea reputedly opens the pores freely and produces sweating. It may be sweetened with honey.

Combined Formulas

Chest Colds. Sometimes a cold may settle in the chest. For this condition the following may be used:

Mix together:
yarrow herb	1 oz.
elder flowers	½ oz.
boneset herb	½ oz.
Spanish licorice	¼ oz.

The mixture is simmered slowly in two pints of water for 20 minutes, then strained. One teacupful is taken three or four times daily, and at bedtime. Solid food is not to be eaten for 24 to 48 hours; fruit juices alone are taken during that period.

Head Colds. Mix together the following:

fluid extract of yarrow	½ ounce
fluid extract of sage	½ ounce
fluid extract of boneset	½ ounces
fluid extract of echinacea	½ ounce

Add water to six fluid ounces. Two teaspoonfuls are taken in a small glass of water, before meals.

Bronchitis. For this condition some European herbalists recommend a three-day fast, followed by a three-day fruit diet. Take an Epsom salts bath once weekly, and deep breathing exercises at least three times daily. The following herbal formula is also used:

Mix thoroughly one ounce each of yarrow, mullein, and elecampane. Place one ounce of the mixture in one pint of cold water and bring to a boil. Simmer slowly for five minutes, then strain. One teacupful is taken every four hours.

Influenza. Herbalists advise going to bed immediately, and drinking plenty of water and fruit juices. No food for 48 hours. The following herbal formula is taken:

One ounce each of yarrow, elder flowers, agrimony, horehound, ground ivy and peppermint are well mixed, then divided into four parts. To one part add two pints of water. Bring to a boil and simmer slowly for 15 minutes, then cool and strain. One-half teacupful is taken warm every two hours.

Catarrh. Mix together one ounce each of yarrow flowers, angelica herb and eyebright herb with a pinch of cinnamon. Place two to three teaspoons of the mixture in a teapot and pour on boiling water. Steep for five minutes, then strain. One teacupful is taken three times daily after each meal.

Accessory Treatment for Catarrh. An herbal consultant in England recommends the following program for catarrh:

The only means of ridding the body of long-standing catarrh is by a strict diet consisting of fresh fruits and vegetables, supplemented by the protein foods such as meat, fish, eggs, cheese, milk, nuts, etc., and if possible compost-grown cereals. If a herbal mixture is taken after each meal, this will assist in neutralizing toxins forming the acids which cause catarrh.

Walking in good country air is of particular benefit to sufferers from this trouble. They should learn to deep-breathe rhythmically and walk for at least two miles a day.

Baths and friction rubs also help to relieve the tissues of waste and poisonous matter, and to tone up the circulation. Try brushing the skin lightly with two small nail brushes, all over the body, to facilitate its work of elimination.

Catarrh does not easily yield to every form of treatment and great will power is required to adhere to diet, herbalism, nature cure, homeopathy, or whichever treatment is selected, until definite results are seen. I have personally known people who have battled with their trouble and persistently kept to a good cleansing diet and routine until they have cleared their bodies of excess acids and cured their catarrh. So with effort it can be done.

The greatest enemy of catarrhal sufferers is white sugar and confectionery of all kinds. This should be replaced by barbados or soft brown sugar. Sweet cakes and biscuits should not be indulged in regularly. Often the fact of giving these up effects a cure by itself.

Smoking is also an irritant if indulged in excessively and is probably the reason why so many young people in their twenties and thirties suffer from catarrh of the chest, nose, and throat.

Milk is not regarded as a good food in these cases and can create an abundance of mucus. It should be taken in minimum quantities only.

In addition to the above program, the herbalist advises taking two garlic perles daily, mid-morning and mid-afternoon.

CHINESE LOQUAT SYRUP

Loquat syrup, a translation of the Chinese language pronunciation of the name "Pei Pa Koa," was originated by Kingto Nin Jiom in the Ching dynasty. This herb formula has a fascinating history. According to the story, Governor Yeung of Peiping (the city where the king lived) was extremely devoted to his mother and terribly grieved because she suffered frequent attacks of painful sore throat and severe coughing spells. Many famous doctors were consulted, but none was able to help.

Then one day Governor Yeung heard of a learned Chinese physician named Yip Tin Sie and immediately engaged him to cure his mother's illnesses. The wise doctor bethought himself of the formula originated by Kingto Nin Jiom and decided to treat her with the herb syrup. After Governor Yeung's mother fully recovered, the doctor gave Governor Yeung the secret formula for the syrup and told him how to prepare it. The governor was further instructed to give his mother some of the syrup twice a day, once in the morning and once in the evening, to maintain her health and to prevent any further recurrence of her ailment.

Governor Yeung was so grateful for his mother's recovery that he prepared bottles of the syrup and gave them away free to anyone who suffered from the same illness.

After the governor's death, the demand for bottles of the syrup became so great that his descendants were forced to charge a little money for them, but to every bottle they attached the complete formula and the mark and words, "Filial to Mother Device," in honor of their ancestors.

Pei Pa Koa Comes to the United States

Loquat Syrup (Pei Pa Koa) contains absolutely no chemicals of any kind. It is a purely natural formula containing eleven herbal ingredients, and it is still prepared in the traditional method.

This syrup, which has been used for centuries in China, is now imported into the United States, and many people are claiming excellent results with its use. One man wrote: "Constant tickle of 'smoker's cough' yielded entirely with the use of Loquat Syrup, and I found the same to be true of an aggravating cough due to a bad cold." A young mother reported that her little boy who suffered from asthma was troubled with coughing spells at night. She said, "I finally tried Loquat Syrup and gave him a teaspoonful one night. It was like a miracle. The coughing soon stopped. After a few nights of doing this, he no longer gets those coughing spells. The syrup has not helped his asthma but what a Godsend it has been with eliminating that terrible coughing."

COLTSFOOT

Botanical Name: *Tussilago farfara*
Common Names: Coughwort, Horse-hoof

This herb grows in fields, ditches, and on the sides of cliffs. The leaves do not appear until after the brilliant yellow flowers have withered. The common name of coltsfoot was given to the herb because of the resemblance of the smooth leaf to that of a colt's foot. The botanical name *Tussilago* signifies "cough dispeller" in reference to the use of the herb as a remedy for pulmonary complaints. In France, coltsfoot was considered so valuable in medicine that the flower could be seen painted on the walls and windows of many pharmacies.

Medicinal Uses

The action of coltsfoot is classed as demulcent, expectorant, and tonic. It is one of the most popular of herbal cough remedies and is also used for other respiratory complaints. The herb is generally given in combination with other specific herbs or natural ingredients. Following are some examples:

For Coughs and Bronchitis

1. Mix one ounce each of coltsfoot, horehound herb, and hyssop. Place one-third of the mixture in one pint of water and bring to a boil. Simmer slowly for ten minutes, then strain. One wineglassful is taken every two hours in acute cases, and three times daily in chronic cases. In stubborn cases a pinch of cayenne pepper is added to the decoction.

2. Mix one ounce of coltsfoot, one-half ounce of elecampane, and one-quarter ounce of marshmallow root. Place the mixture in two pints of water, boil slowly for 15 minutes, then cool and strain. One wineglassful is taken three times daily.
3. Mix together one ounce each of coltsfoot, horehound, violet leaves, and marshmallow root. Place one-quarter of the mixture in one and one-half pints of water. Boil down to one pint. Strain and sweeten with honey. The decoction may be taken in teacupful doses as frequently as desired.

Asthma and Colds. Boil one ounce of coltsfoot leaves in one quart of water down to one pint, then strain. Add one teaspoonful of honey. The decoction is taken frequently in teacupful doses.

ANISE

Botanical Name: *Pimpinella anisum*
Common Name: Anise

Anise is native to Egypt, Greece, and Asia Minor, but is cultivated and grown commercially in many parts of the world. In the East, in former times, anise was used with other spices as part payment of taxes. In Germany, it is used to flavor cakes and soups. It is largely employed in Spain, Italy, France, and South America in the preparation of cordial liqueurs.

Medicinal Action and Uses

The action of anise is classified as pectoral and carminative. It is considered very valuable as a remedy for hard dry cough where expectoration is difficult. For this purpose it is generally used in the form of lozenges.

The volatile oil of anise forms part of the preparation for the liqueur anisette which reputedly is helpful for bronchitis and spasmodic asthma. If anisette is administered in hot water, it is said to be an immediate palliative. (Anisette is easily obtained, being sold in most liquor stores.)

Five drops of anise oil (obtained from herb firms) placed on top of a small amount of honey in a teaspoon taken orally one-half hour before meals has reportedly proved helpful in some cases of emphysema.

HONEY

Among Asiatic races honey is considered excellent for coughs, bronchitis, and other pulmonary complaints. Honey is also a popular home remedy among the Greeks, Italians, and Hungarians.

For respiratory ailments honey is often mixed with anise, ginger, or garlic. A tablespoon of honey added to a glassful of warm milk is used for bronchitis. Five parts of honey to one part of alum mixed in one quart of water is valued as a gargle for sore throat and ulceration of the mouth and gums. One tablespoon of honey with some lemon juice in a glassful of hot water is used to treat influenza.

There are many reports that honey will relieve hay fever and sinus trouble. For these conditions two teapoons of honey are taken at each meal.

Some years ago, Dr. McGrew of El Paso, Texas, stated that during a hay-fever season 33 sufferers of hay fever obtained partial or complete relief by eating honey produced in their area.

TIGER BALM

This is a popular Oriental herbal ointment developed more than half a century ago by two Chinese brothers. The product comes packed in three sizes—large jars, medium jars, and small tins. It also comes in two strengths—mild and strong.

Tiger balm is used for relieving tightness of the chest and for its soothing effect on muscular aches and pains due to colds and exposure. For such conditions, the afflicted parts are well rubbed with the Chinese herbal ointment two or three times daily, and covered with a warm flannel.

Tiger balm is also employed as an inhalant for stuffed-up noses, nasal drip, and head colds. A few whiffs of the vapor soothes the upper air passages and gives the head a clear feeling.

Chinese Tiger Balm is available from various herb firms and health food stores.

GARLIC

Botanical Name: *Allium sativum*
Common Name: Common Garlic

Miraculous healing power appears to exist in the common

garlic. Research shows that for over 5000 years garlic has been used to treat many ailments that are being studied today in modern scientific laboratories. The Babylonians, Chinese, Greeks, Romans, Egyptians, and others knew of its curative power.

Dioscorides, a Greek physician of the second century who accompanied the Roman armies as their official physician, specified garlic for all lung and intestinal disorders occurring among the soldiers.

In Marseilles, a garlic-vinegar preparation known as the *Four Thieves* was credited with protecting many of the people when a plague struck that city (1722). Some claim that the preparation originated with four thieves who confessed they used it with complete protection against the plague while they robbed the bodies of the dead. Others claimed that a man named Richard Forthave developed and sold the preparation, and that the remedy was originally referred to as "Forthave's." However, with the passing of time his surname became corrupted to *Four Thieves*.

In Bulgaria there is a surprising number of people who reach the age of 100 who are still active and working. In that country it is a common practice among the ordinary people to chew garlic regularly.

Some time ago Professor G. Tallarico wrote: "Lakhovsky [an electrobiologist] relates marvels of garlic and the onions because of their content of elements and specific essences. He says that in certain forests of Siberia a variety of wild garlic grows, called locally 'ceremissa.' Every autumn there is a pilgrimage to those forests when the aged, the paralyzed, the sick, and those afflicted with all kinds of disease repair there to eat of the wild garlic for days, or even weeks. Afterward they return to their homes relieved of their ills, rejuvenated and healed. It is further said that in Russia and Poland there are groups of very pious and very poor Israelites who from time to time interrupt their religious exercises to break their fast upon bread and raw garlic. Cancer is unknown among those people, whose life span averages better than a century."

Garlic for Respiratory Disorders

W. T. Fernie, M.D., wrote:

Garlic proves useful in asthma, whooping cough and other spasmodic affections of the chest. For an adult, one or more cloves may be eaten at a time. The odor of the bulb is very diffusible, even when it is applied to the soles of the feet its odor is exhaled by the lungs.

Dr. Bowles, a noted English physician of former times, made use of garlic with much success as a secret remedy for asthma. He concocted a preserve from the boiled cloves with vinegar and sugar, to be kept in an earthen jar. The dose was a bulb or two with some of the syrup, each morning when fasting.

Professor E. Roos of Germany stated: "In recent times, garlic has been highly recommended in France, particularly as a remedy in the case of lung disease attended by copious and ill-smelling expectoration, as well as a remedy against hypertension."

Dr. J. Klosa, another Germany physician, experimented with garlic as a treatment for colds and reported his findings. He used a specially prepared solution of garlic oil and water, which was administered in doses of 10 to 25 drops every four hours. He reports the results with grippe, sore throat, and rhinitis (clogged and running nose) patients. The fever and catarrhal symptoms of 13 cases of grippe were cut short in every case.

In 28 cases of sore throat, the burning and tickling effect abated to a point of disappearance in 24 hours. If caught in its first stages, it was found that further development of sore throat could be halted completely by administering about 30 drops, or about two doses of the oil of garlic solution.

In 71 cases of clogged and running nose, the oil was taken partly by mouth and partly by being administered directly into the nostrils. In 13 to 20 minutes, the nasal congestion was completely cleared up in all cases and there were no further complications.

Another Physician Reports on the Value of Garlic

Kristine Nolfi, M.D., of Denmark, wrote of the value of garlic for various ailments. Here are a few excerpts:

If one puts a piece of garlic in his mouth at the onset of a cold, on both sides between cheek and teeth, the cold will disappear within a few hours or, at most, within a day.

At "Humlegaarden" [Danish health resort] epidemic colds are unknown. Everyone knows that he must use garlic when a cold begins. Since a cold may develop into pneumonia in the case of weak patients, it is better avoided.

A manufacturer from Bergen in Norway, who has been at Humlegaarden several times, was visited one day by a farmer who had a very bad cold. The manufacturer gave him a handful of garlic and told him how to use it. Two days later the farmer telephoned to say that his whole family was well again—their colds had disappeared.

Garlic has also a curative effect on chronic diseases in the upper respiratory organs provided one keeps garlic in his mouth day and night (not while sleeping), renewing the cloves every morning and evening after they have absorbed the poisons. This applies to chronic inflammation of the tonsils, salivary glands and neighboring lymph glands, empyema of the maxillary sinus, severe pharyngitis and laryngitis, bronchitis, and tuberculosis of the lungs.

Garlic—a Potent Germ Killer

One of the known ingredients responsible for the power of garlic as an anti-infection agent is *allinin*. Wallace E. Harrel, M.D., reported that he found *allinin* inhibited growth in large numbers of Gram-positive and Gram-negative microbes. Other scientists have also recognized the anti-bacterial power of garlic.

Investigations by Russian medical researchers have made garlic oil so popular in their country that it is referred to as "Russian Penicillin."

Case History Using Garlic Tablets

According to many people, garlic in tablet form has proved valuable for treating certain respiratory ailments. For example: Mrs. C.L.T. of South Wales writes: "Garlic tablets cured me of a virus infection of the chest earlier this year. After 14 weeks on antibiotics which did nothing to help, the garlic brought quick results. After two weeks I was a different person. I have sent for more as a precaution against colds. I thought you'd like to know about this."

OTHER METHODS OF USING GARLIC

1. As an inhalant for nasal congestion, a little chopped garlic and one teaspoon of vinegar are placed in a container of hot water. The fumes are inhaled through the nose, and repeated as often as necessary.
2. Garlic tea may be used for stubborn coughs and colds and also to relieve sinus congestion. Two to four freshly

chopped garlic cloves are added to one quart of water brought to a boil. As soon as the water boils it is immediately removed from the burner and allowed to steep as ordinary tea, then strained. One hot teacupful is sipped slowly three or four times a day. if the cough or cold is very severe the tea may be used every hour until relief is obtained.

3. For asthma, bronchitis, sore throat, colds and coughs, the freshly expressed juice of garlic is mixed well with honey and a teaspoonful of the mixture taken at repeated intervals.

4. Garlic taken daily in tablet or capsule form is another method credited with fighting various respiratory ailments.

5. For tonsillitis, one tablespoon of fresh garlic juice and two ounces of sage are placed in a covered container with one quart of water and brought to a boil. As soon as the water boils, the container is immediately removed from the burner and the tea allowed to stand until lukewarm, then strained. One small teacupful is taken four or five times a day. In addition, another quart or more of the garlic-sage tea is prepared in the same way, and used as a hot gargle, about one cupful every half-hour until relief is obtained.

NATURAL PROGRAM FOR TREATING HAY FEVER

Dr. Jon Evans of England presents the following information and treatment for alleviating the condition of hay fever:[6]

Although most of us look to the summer months with pleasure, there are still those who dread this time of year. They anticipate, and indeed are often inflicted with, a personal purgatory—that distressing complaint commonly known as hay fever.

This highly sensitized state of the mucous membranes of the nose and bronchial tubes is nearly always produced by a toxic condition of long standing. When the lining membranes are affected they become congested; the sufferer breathes in quickly but cannot expire air properly, and is shaken by a tormenting cough and choking sensation or a paroxysm of sneezing which produces copious tears. It is quite common for urticarial rashes consisting of wheals and red spots or patches to appear on the body at the same time.

---

[6]*Health from Herbs*, September–October 1968.

Many practitioners will have noticed that with hay fever sufferers, apart from sneezing, tightness in the chest and the other symptoms already mentioned, there is a general disposition towards lassitude with depression.

When the membranes of the nasal organ become highly sensitive it is easy to see why the summer should be the worst period for people addicted to hay fever. The pollen and tiny particles of grass and plants settle in the nasal passages and bronchial tubes, thus causing irritation.

Allopathic treatment is, in the main, suppressive; at its best it will alleviate the symptoms. Ephedrine tablets are often prescribed for use during an attack; the drug may also be given in the form of a spray; sometimes adrenalin is provided as a means of treatment. Such action is useless and can be dangerous. The patient is never without an "inhaler" or drugs and is certainly no further towards a cure.

It has been discovered that in many patients suffering from hay fever there is a deficiency of Vitamin A; it is therefore essential that the diet be carefully balanced. Carrot juice is one of the richest sources of Vitamin A and the body can assimilate it easily. Apart from carrots, this particular vitamin is to be found in kale, parsley, turnip greens, broccoli, dandelion leaves, endive and watermelon. I invariably include a variety of natural foods rich in Vitamin A in the patient's diet. Obviously the intake of starchy and sugary substances must be drastically reduced; no white sugar or white bread; pastries and chocolate definitely out.

Practitioners who prescribe juice therapy will find the following formula very effective in the treatment of hay fever. I am quite sure that if they advise their patients to adhere to the correct diet, juice therapy and any necessary herbal prescriptions, the predisposing factors causing the complaint will be quickly eliminated.

In all, 16 ounces of juice should be taken daily; any one of the three combinations can be used.

(1) Carrot 8 oz., celery 8 oz.
(2) Carrot 6 oz., beet 5 oz., cucumber 5 oz.
(3) Carrot 8 oz., celery 4 oz., spinach 2 oz., parsley 2 oz.

If the household is fortunate enough to own an electric juicer, all kinds of fruits and vegetables can be used for making vital health drinks. An investment in such a piece of kitchen equipment will prove invaluable.

Having dealt briefly with the dietary aspects, we must now consider appropriate herbal medication. Remember we treat the patient as a whole and not merely the symptoms.

The two prescriptions which I am recommending have proved

highly successful and I have no hesitation in commending their use.

#1   Chamomile .... ½ oz.
      Horehound herb .... ½ oz.
      Bayberry Bark ..... ½ oz.
      Eyebright .... ½ oz.

Cover the herbs with two pints of water. Bring slowly to the boil, simmer for 10 minutes, remove and allow to stand for 30 minutes, stirring from time to time. Strain; one cupful, in sips, three times a day.

#2   Fluid Extract Wood Betony .... 4 drachms*
      "   "   Yarrow .... 8 drachms
      "   "   Eyebright .... 6 drachms
      "   "   Capsicum .... 10 drops
                     Water, to 8 oz.

Dose: Three teaspoonfuls in a wineglass of water, three times a day after meals.

Both the prescriptions contain that sovereign remedy Eyebright, which acts specifically on the mucous lining of the eyes and nose, also the upper part of the throat. Hay fever, acute attacks of cold in the head, and troublesome symptoms due to catarrh often respond to a simple infusion of Eyebright alone (one ounce to one pint of boiling water). A wineglass of the infusion to be taken four or five times a day. This herb has been in medical use for centuries—in the main for disorders of the eyes. It was recommended as far back as 1329 by Matthaeus Sylvaticus, a physician who wrote a treatise on its virtues.

SUMMARY

1. Specific herbs and herbal products are natural remedies for coping with a large variety of respiratory ailments.

2. Centuries of experience in many parts of the world have confirmed that herbal remedies help fight infection, loosen stubborn phlegm, reduce fever, soothe irritated air passages and lungs, and help bring an end to dragged-out respiratory miseries.

3. External herbal applications relieve chest tightness and muscular aches and pains due to colds.

4. Specific herbal preparations may be used as inhalants for

---

*One drachm equals approximately one teaspoonful.

coping with nasal congestion, nasal drip, head colds, and similar conditions.

5. Herb gargles, fomentations, and poultices are helpful accessory treatments for various respiratory conditions.

CHAPTER 5

Herbs for Urinary Complaints

There are a multitude of herbs used in various parts of the world for urinary disorders. Under the circumstances, space will not permit a complete coverage; therefore let us consider some of the most popular, and the urinary ailments for which they are used.

UVA-URSI

Botanical Name: *Arctostaphylos uva-ursi*
Common Name: Bearberry

This small evergreen shrub grows in Europe, Asia, and North America. Although the bright red berries produced by the plant are tasteless and dry, they formed an important article of diet among the North American Indians. They received their common name of Bearberry because bears were very fond of the fruit. In the eastern part of the country, the Indians called the plant *Kinnikinnick*.

Uva-ursi has a longstanding reputation as a remedy of great value in disease of the bladder and kidneys, and as tonic to the urinary organs. Records shows that it was used by Welsh physicians in the 13th century. It was recommended for medicinal use in Germany in 1763, and was included in the *London Pharmacopeia* for the first time in 1788. Among the many herbs used by the Indians as diuretics to increase the flow of urine, uva-ursi was regarded as the outstanding remedy.

Modern Medicinal Use

Uva-ursi contains a glycoside called *arbutin* and owes much of its marked diuretic action to this substance. During the excretion by the kidneys, *arbutin* exercises an antiseptic effect on the urinary mucous membrane. Uva-ursi is therefore considered to be of value in various conditions of the urinary tract such as cystitis, urethritis, and so on. Uva-ursi is also said to be a strengthener of the sphincter muscle, and as such is useful in conditions of "night rising" and incontinence. For this particular purpose, the herb is used alone, and prepared as an instant tea—one teasponful of the powdered herb to one cup of boiling water. One cup of the tea is taken every morning and evening.

For cystitis, the following combined formula is used: uva-ursi leaves, half an ounce; peach leaves, half an ounce; gravel root (*Eupatorium purpureum*), one ounce; clivers herb, one ounce; wintergreen leaves, a quarter of an ounce. The herbs are thoroughly mixed together and boiled slowly in four pints of water for 10 minutes, then strained. It is taken in half teacupful doses four or five times daily.

For relieving conditions of urethritis, gravel, stones, scalding urine, and various other bladder and kidney complaints, uva-ursi is combined with other select herbs and prepared and used as follows:

One ounce each of uva-ursi, clivers, juniper berries, buchu, parsley piert, sage and marshmallow leaves are pulverized, then mixed thoroughly and stored in a capped jar. One teaspoonful of the mixture is placed in a cup and boiling water added. The cup is covered with a saucer, and the tea allowed to stand for 10 minutes, then strained. One cup of the tea is taken three times daily (once before each meal). In more stubborn cases one cup is taken every three hours. If necessary, another supply of the herb mixture may be prepared and stored in a jar for further use.

A medical herbalist of England recommends the following treatment for the condition of cystitis:[1]

At the onset of an attack, go to bed and avoid chills. Regulate the diet. Give plenty of vegetables. Milk and fish are suitable. Drink plenty of barley water and dandelion coffee. Avoid starchy

---

[1]*Health from Herbs*, November 1953.

foods, sweets and meats, also ordinary coffee and alcohol. Bathe frequently. Get the following herbs finely cut, and make an infusion:

Uva-ursi .... 3 parts
Kava kava .... 3 parts
Hydrangea .... 3 parts
Marshmallow leaves .... 3 parts
Buchu .... 1 part
Parsley priert .... 3 parts

Mix well and divide into four parts. To one part add a pint of boiling water. Cool, strain, and take half a teacupful three times daily between meals.

SEVEN BARKS

Botanical Name: *Hydrangea arborescens*
Common Name: Seven Barks

Hydrangea is known by the common name of seven barks because the bark peels off in separate layers of different colors. The botanical name is from *hydro* (water), and *angeion* (a vessel), in reference to the cuplike form of the capsule or seed vessel. However, some say that this name was given because hydrangea is a marsh plant and requires lots of water.

Seven barks was an old Cherokee Indian remedy used for disorders of the urinary system. It was first brought to the attention of the medical profession in 1850 by Dr. S. W. Butler, whose father, a physician and missionary, had lived among the Cherokees and used the root of this plant with considerable advantage in treating calculi complaints. Later its value in these conditions was confirmed by Drs. Atlee D. Horsely and John S. C. Monkur. Dr. Butler employed it either as a regular decoction or as a syrup by mixing honey or sugar with the decoction.

Early in the twentieth century, physicians who wrote books on home remedies invariably cited seven barks as a valuable healing agent. For example, the following is a typical write-up of the remedy from those times:

Hydrangea: Seven barks
Part Used: The root
It is an admirable remedy for gravel, and relieves that excruciating pain experienced when the gravelly formations pass through the ureters from the kidney to the bladder. Its curative qualities for inflammation of the kidney, as well as other affections of the

urinary organs, are now generally recognized ... Dose of the decoction, one teaspoonful several times a day.

In modern Europe, medical herbalists regard the plant as a valuable tonic for the bladder and kidneys. It reputedly has a mild but permanent tonic effect, dissolves calculus, eliminates pain, and subdues inflammation. It is also highly valued abroad for its power of preventing the formation of gravelly deposits.

Case History

A woman, the mother of 12 children, was seriously ill, passing blood. The doctor told the family that she had only a few days to live. A neighbor happened to drop by and when he told the stricken family that seven barks would heal the mother, the father replied that he had not the slightest idea where he might find the plant. The neighbor quickly informed him that his farm was full of it. Small amounts of the decoction, made by boiling one ounce of the root in one pint of boiling water, were carefully dripped into the mouth of the semi-conscious woman, who was gently nudged so that she could manage to swallow it. In a few days, much to the astonishment of the doctor and the family, the woman was well. She wrote an article about her experience, which was published in the forum of a newspaper, and before long she received over 400 letters inquiring about seven barks. For 15 years the family dug and mailed hundreds of packages of the root until they finally sold the farm.

PARSLEY

Botanical Name: *Apium petroselinum*
Common Name: Garden Parsley

Parsley is extremely rich in vitamins A and C. It also contains iron, calcium, phosphorus, manganese, potassium, and vitamin B_1. In addition to its vitamin and mineral content, it contains mucilage, sugar, starch, volatile oil, and *apiol*. The herb is classified medicinally as diuretic, aperient, and emmenagogue. it is reputed to act as a solvent for uric acid when used as a tea or eaten after meals.

R. D. Pope, M.D., has done considerable research on this plant and says that it is "excellent for the genito-urinary tract, of great assistance in the calculi of the kidneys and bladder, albuminaria, nephritis and other kidney trouble. It has properties essential to oxygen metabolism and in maintaining normal action of the adrenal and thyroid glands."

One doctor who made a trip to Holland was surprised to find that the people there were using parsley tea with very good effect for urinary trouble and prostate pressure. When he returned from his trip he began recommending parsley tea to his patients.

How to Prepare the Tea

Parsley tea is prepared by placing a fresh bunch of parsley in a saucepan and adding two pints of cold water. This is brought to a boil and simmered not more than ten seconds. The vessel is then covered, removed from the burner, allowed to stand until cold, and then strained. Four to five cups of the tea are taken daily until results are obtained. (The cold tea may be reheated and taken warm.)

Although the leaves of parsley are the part of the herb most commonly used to prepare the tea, the beverage may be made from the dried roots if one prefers. In this case, a heaping tablespoonful of the dried cut roots is boiled slowly in one quart of water for 15 minutes. The decoction is allowed to stand until cold, then strained and taken in cupful doses four times daily.

If the fluid extract of the root is used, one-half to one teaspoonful is taken in a little water three times daily.

PARSLEY PIERT

Botanical Name: *Alchemilla arvensis*
Common Name: Parsley Breakstone

This common little plant is widely distributed throughout Europe, North Africa, and North America. Parsley piert is not related to the common parsley; however, its medicinal action is somewhat similar. It has an astringent taste but no odor, and is classified as diuretic, demulcent, and refrigerant. In olden times the herb was called "parsley breakstone," and to this day the plant has retained its reputation as an effective remedy for gravel, kidney and bladder stones, and other urinary complaints. Several London physicians prescribe this remedy regularly. The infusion is taken in teacupful doses three times daily. Of the liquid extract, one teaspoonful in a small glass of water is taken twice a day.

Although parsley piert forms a useful remedy when taken alone, medical herbalists state that it is even more effective when combined with other diuretics, such as pellitory-of-the-wall, buchu leaves, gravelroot, wild carrot, juniper berries, or parsley root. And to sooth and assist the passage of an irritating substance, a demulcent such as marshmallow, comfrey or slippery elm bark is often included in the combined formula.

Either of the following mixtures can be given for stone in the bladder, gravel, and all urinary troubles when deposits are present:

- Parsley piert 1 oz.; pellitory-of-the-wall 1 oz.; wild carrot 1 oz.; buchu ½ oz. The herbs are mixed together and divided into three portions. One portion is added to one pint of boiling water, and allowed to stand for 15 minutes, then strained. One wineglassful is taken four times daily.
- Mix together one-half ounce each of parsley piert, pellitory-of-the-wall, gravel root, and one ounce of marshmallow root. Boil in two and a half pints of water down to two pints. Cool, strain, and take a wineglassful three times daily.

HORSETAIL

Botanical Name: *Equisetum arvense*
Common Names: Shave Grass, Scouring Rush, Dutch Rush

This is a perennial plant which grows in sand and gravel along roadsides, and in damp, wet places. The botanical name *Equisetum* is derived from the Latin words *equus* (a horse) and *seta* (a bristle), from the odd bristly appearance of the jointed stems of the plant. Because of this appearance it has been given the popular name of horsetail.

Constituents and Uses

Horsetail is rich in minerals, especially silica. It is regarded by European herbalists as a grand remedy for urinary complaints, e.g., gravel, inflammation of the urinary passages, cystitis, and weakness of the kidneys and bladder. It is also reputed to be very effective for lack of bladder control such as bed wetting in children and incontinence (inability to hold the urine) in older people.

The infusion is prepared by pouring one pint of boiling water over one ounce of the herb. The tea is allowed to stand until cold, then taken in tablespoonful doses before meals. If the tincture is used, ½ to one teaspoonful is taken in a little water two or three times daily.

NOTE: Herbalists advise that for conditions of bed wetting, no fluids should be taken after 5 P.M., except a very minimum of plain water in case of thirst.

BUCKWHEAT HONEY

Buckwheat honey is another of the various remedies used for bed wetting. From one teaspoonful to one tablespoonful taken at bedtime has proved effective in many cases.

KIDNEY BEAN PODS
(A Rediscovered Remedy)

Botanical Name: *Phaseolus vulgaris*
Common Name: Kidney Bean

According to Captain Frank Roberts, a medical herbalist of England, permanent cures of disorders of the kidneys and urinary bladder have been achieved with a decoction of kidney bean pods. The remedy was accidentally discovered by Dr. Ramm of Preetz in Holstein, Germany. Back in 1881, he was treating a female patient for dropsy following a valvular disease of the heart. Then suddenly the patient disappeared, but sometime afterwards while making his rounds he happened to meet her and was surprised to find that she showed no signs of dropsy.

She explained to Dr. Ramm that she had been using various herbal teas and that one day she had accidentally drunk a tumblerful of kidney bean pod water, thinking it was a new herbal infusion she had prepared. Shortly after drinking it, she began passing tremendous quantities of urine. To make certain that it was not just a coincidence, she took another tumblerful of the bean pod water, and again vast quantities of water were voided, all of it as clear as crystal.

She continued taking the decoction and within three weeks she no longer had any sign whatsoever of dropsy. She kept on with the bean pod water for another couple of weeks and then stopped. From that time on she was healthy, and there had been no further return of the disease.

Dr. Ramm was completely fascinated. He prepared the bean

pod water and began prescribing and dispensing it for every type of urinary disease that came to his attention.

A Remarkable Diuretic

Dr. Ramm also determined to discover any other possible uses for this remarkable remedy. First it was given to every dropsy case he had under treatment. Then he used it for all heart cases that tended toward dropsy. In every case, large quantities of clear urine were voided. The doctor found that even the most advanced longstanding dropsies were dispersed and remained cured after only a few days on the decoction.

The doctor learned that the large quantities of albumin in the urine soon grew less and vanished upon the cure of the dropsical condition, and did not recur after discontinuation of the treatment.

Other Ailments Corrected

As Dr. Ramm's research went on, further gratifying results were obtained. It was found that chronic albuminous conditions of the kidneys responded to the kidney bean pod water treatment. Hemorrhage from any part of the urinary tract was quickly arrested. Kidney inflammations and various chronic kidney diseases were corrected.

Small kidney stones and gravel were quickly dissolved, and here again the doctor noted the absence of any tendency for the condition to recur after completion of treatment. Diseases of the bladder and ureters were also cured.

Acute and chronic gout yielded to this decoction. However, in cases of gout, rheumatism, and large kidney stones, Dr. Ramm found that the decoction worked slowly and had to be used with perseverance.

In all the diseases treated, the patient encountered no relapse if two or three glassfuls of the bean pod water were taken every week.

Diabetes

The use of bean pod water in diabetes showed that traces of sugar vanished from the urine in three or four weeks. A strict diabetic diet was adhered to during the three or four weeks of treatment.

Dr. Ramm reported cases of diabetic patients who had taken

treatment 12 years previously and had failed to take occasional drinks of the decoction and still had no sign of a return of the disease. Others had experienced a slight return of sugar in the urine after a lapse of time without the remedy, and these had quickly put things right with a few glassfuls of the kidney bean pod water.

Remedy Given by Enema

In some cases the remedy was found to cause vomiting or other adverse conditions. For these cases, Dr. Ramm administered the decoction by enema in quantities of half a pint mixed with a saltspoonful of salt every two or four fours. The results were just as favorable as if taken by mouth. He also found that the enema would halt the convulsions of uremia (urinary constituents in the blood) and produce copious diuresis just as effectively as the decoction did when taken by mouth.

Freshness of Remedy Essential

When Dr. Ramm eventually published a report on his research, he stressed the fact that only *freshly* prepared kidney bean pod water contained the potent medicinal qualities. He insisted that results could be expected only if the freshly made bean pod water was taken the same day it was prepared.

How to Prepare the Remedy

There is a limited period of the year when fresh kidney bean pods are available. They will have to be grown in your garden, or if you have no such facilities you may be able to grow them in a friend's garden.

To prepare the remedy, Dr. Ramm advised that you pick the bean pods when ripe, and immediately make the decoction from the sliced pods *without the beans.* (The potency of the remedy lies in the *pods*, not in the beans.) Put two ounces of the bean pods in four quarts of hot water and boil slowly for four hours. Remove from the burner, let cool, then strain the liquid through a fine muslin cloth into a container. Put in the refrigerator for about eight hours. Since the decoction must be drunk within 24 hours of picking the pods, if it is prepared at bedtime it will stand during the eight hours of sleep.

After allowing the decoction to stand for eight hours, pour the remedy, without stirring it, through another clean piece of muslin. Try to disturb the sediment as little as possible. The more carefully this is done the less likely it is that any intestinal disturbance will occur during treatment. The decoction is then ready for use. It should not be taken after a lapse of 24 hours as it will cause severe diarrhea and will have no curative effect on the urinary disorder. One glassful of the decoction is taken every two hours throughout the day. If these instructions are followed, Dr. Ramm reports that the remedy is completely safe and can be taken indefinitely.

Another Doctor's Findings

About the same time Dr. Ramm published his paper on the kidney bean pod remedy, Dr. Isenburg of Hamburg, Germany, confirmed its curative power. One of Dr. Isenburg's patients reports as follows:

About nine years ago, in 1897, I began to suffer from a very disagreeable feeling of pressure in the region of the bladder, which increased to an intense pain through excitement or psychic depression. In the course of the next years this state very slowly became worse, until in 1906 violent pains appeared in the right ureter. At the same time the pain in the bladder suddenly increased considerably. My physician diagnosed an inflammation of both organs, but none of all those I consulted were able to give me any relief.

The urine showed pus, sometimes in considerable quantity. In 1905, some time before these last symptoms developed, others had appeared which consisted of severe pains in the back in the neck. They tormented me constantly, and often I could not fall asleep. Cold rubs and liniments brought only a temporary improvement.

The pains constantly increased in the spring of 1906 and muscular rheumatism set in. This was so violent that I could hardly wash myself in the morning and evening. Rubbings with water and plasters hardly brought any relief. These various ailments finally became so very bad that I was never free from pain; and they increased constantly in violence.

At this time—in the summer of 1906—the tea of ripe bean pods was recommended to me, and my attention was called to the pamphlet of Dr. Ramm of Preetz, in Holstein. So I sent for five pounds of the bean pods. ("It was found that the ripe bean pods could be picked and kept for some time before being prepared. This only applied to the pods when ripe," according to Frank Roberts.)

I began the treatment according to directions. I did not have to wait long for results; large masses of uric acid crystals and albuminous matter were excreted, and that initiated a decrease of the pain in the bladder and kidneys. The pain in the bladder disappeared entirely in about three weeks; the muscular rheumatism also diminished in the next few weeks to disappear entirely in seven or eight weeks.

I was soon entirely free from my very great sufferings and have not had any trouble since, as I have been using the tea off and on. The enormous excretion of uric acid crystals during the use of the tea was really remarkable (they often covered the bottom of the night vessel).

Concluding Remarks

In conclusion, medical herbalist Frank Roberts says of the remedy: "It has already been prescribed in many cases. Without going into details, I can assure you it never fails."

NOTE: If taken as directed, the kidney bean pod water should be completely harmless, as Dr. Ramm has stated. Nevertheless, if you should decide to use it, it would be best to start with just small quantities, about a half a glass a day. That amount would not have any therapeutic effect but might indicate if you are subject to any possible adverse effect. Only when you are certain you are not sensitive to the decoction should you attempt using it.

MARSHMALLOW

Botanical Name: *Althea officinalis*
Common Name: Sweet Weed

Marshmallow is a perennial herb with pale purplish flowers, and grows on the borders of salt marshes, in damp meadows, and on the banks of tidal rivers. The generic name, Althea, is taken from the Greek, *altho*, meaning "to cure," in reference to its healing properties.

Marshmallow has been used both as a food and a remedy since the very earliest periods. Records show that Charlemagne (742–814 A.D.) demanded that it be cultivated in his domain. Among the Romans a dish of marshmallow was considered a delicacy. Many of the poorer people of Syria subsisted for weeks on various herbs of which marshmallow was one of the most popular. Because of the plant's soothing qualities, Arab physicians in early times prepared the leaves as a poultice to relieve inflammation. Dioscorides and other herbalists of olden times praised the herb as a valuable and useful remedy.

Modern Uses

M. Bacon discovered a principle in marshmallow root which is identical with *asparagin*. Marshmallow also contains pectin, starch, bassorin, tannin, and phosphates. Its therapeutic action is classified as demulcent, emollient, and mucilaginous.

Because of its soothing and healing therapeutic properties, marshmallow root is extensively employed in Europe as a remedy in irritation and inflammation of the alimentary and genito-urinary system. French druggists use the powdered root in the preparation of electuaries and pills. In France the tender leaves and young tops are eaten uncooked, in spring salads, for their property of stimulating the kidneys. A syrup made from the root is used for the same purposes. The herb is also considered a good remedy for scalding urine, cystitis, and other urinary complaints.

A decoction of marshmallow is prepared by placing four ounces of the dried roots into five pints of water and boiling down to three pints. This is strained, and drunk freely.

If the leaves are used, the tea is prepared as an ordinary infusion.

Case History

With reference to the value of marshmallow, Dr. Bartram writes:[2] "Mrs. S.C.M. of Southport found it worked like a charm on her painful cystitis. Unable to get the root, she placed two to three heaped teaspoonfuls of the dried leaves into a small enamel saucepan and covered with a teacupful of cold water. This she brought to the boil and simmered for half a minute. Setting it aside until cold, she strained it and drank a wineglassful after meals three times daily. She was more than pleased when she found a nasty, raw condition of her mouth also cleared up."

Combined Formula

A woman consulted a European herbalist, explaining that whenever her young son became upset, he started to wet the bed. She said the condition lasted a week, a month, or even longer,

---

[2]*Health from Herbs*, September–October 1969.

and that nearly everything had been tried without permanent benefit. She added, "I should so like to have him free from this weakness before he starts going away to school."

The herbalist recommended the following formula:

Fluid extract of marshmallow one-half ounce, fluid extract of agrimony one ounce; fluid extract of buchu one-half ounce; fluid extract of licorice root one drachm (approx. one teaspoon). Mix the extracts together and add water to six ounces. Dose: One dessertspoonful in water three times daily. Regulate the dose according to age. Or give three drops of Mullein Oil on sugar or with honey three times daily. For those over 12 years old, the dose is five drops.

PIPSISSEWA

Botanical Name: *Chimaphila umbellata*
Common Names: Prince's Pine, Ground Holly

This is a small evergreen shrub with a creeping rhizome. It bears flowers of a light purple color which emit a fragrant aroma. This plant grows in Europe, Asia, Siberia, and is found in all parts of the United States.

Certain Indian tribes prepared a tea made with pipsissewa and employed it for a variety of genito-urinary disorders such as nephritis, chronic cystitis, and urethritis. It was also used for rheumatism and to reestablish the menstrual flow after childbirth. The remedy passed from the hands of the Indians to those of the early settlers, where it retained its popularity for years before being adopted by the medical profession.

The leaves of pipsissewa were scientifically examined as early as 1860 by Fairbanks who found that they contain starch, sugar, pectic acid, resin, tannic acid, fatty matter, chlorophyll, lignin, a yellowish coloring matter, and a substance which he called *chimaphillin*.

Recent scientific research with a plant has shown that it possesses antibacterial power. The alcoholic and water extracts have been found to contain *in vitro* antibiotic activity. Two hundred and nine Nova Scotian plants were tested for antibacterial power against *E. coli* and *Staph aureus* by Bishop and MacDonald. Pipsissewa was reported to be one of the ten most active plants.

Modern herbalists classify the medicinal action of pipsissewa as astringent, tonic, diuretic, and alternative. It is reputed to be of much value for bladder and kidney problems, and a good remedy for ascites. One teaspoon of the herb is placed in a cup and boiling water is added. The cup is covered with a saucer and allowed to steep for ten minutes, then strained. One cup of the tea is taken three times daily. If the tincture is used, one-half to one teaspoonful is taken in a small glass of water three times a day.

CHINESE SUPER OLD-FASHIONED COMPOUND HERB TEA

This is a special Chinese formula consisting of several herbs, processed, compounded, and prepared as a tea by a traditional method. For thousands of years the Chinese people of the Heung San district in China have used the herb tea for relieving or preventing various ailments of the urinary system, such as kidney obstructions by albuminous conditions, inflammatory disorders of the bladder and kidneys, certain diseases of the ureter and urethra, and so on. The tea reportedly also dissolves or removes those many small painful kidney stones and gravel which so many people tend to develop. And Chinese men have long used this ancient herb compound to prevent or relieve prostate trouble. (See chapter on men's ailments.)

Chinese Super Old-Fashioned Compound Herb Tea comes already prepared in liquid form packed in bottles. There are three strengths. The regular is called "Fancy"; the stronger comes in a two-bottle set called "Super 1" and "Super 2." The Fancy also comes in powdered form contained in capsules.

How the Fancy Compound Is Used

According to the Chinese, the Fancy herb compound produces a cleansing and healing effect on the urinary organs and passages. It is easy to use. First the bottle of tea is well shaken; then the tea is poured into a porcelain or enamel pot. The pot is covered with a lid and the tea heated until warm enough to drink. It is taken on an empty stomach.

One bottle of the Fancy tea is used once every day until the ailment has cleared up; then one bottle may be taken once a month or every other month thereafter as a preventative measure against any recurrence of the problem.

Many Chinese people who have never been troubled by any type of urinary ailment drink one bottle of the Fancy compound tea every month, claiming that it acts as a preventative against ever gettting such disorders.

If the capsules of the Fancy in powdered form are used, they are taken according to the directions on the bottle.

Super 1 and Super 2

For more stubborn urinary problems, the Chinese use the stronger strengths of the compound tea. The treatment requires the two-bottle set, which consists of one large bottle and one small, called respectively Chinese Super 1 Old-Fashioned Compound Herb Tea and Chinese Super 2 Old-Fashioned Compound Herb Tea.

After the bottle has been shaken well, the Super 1 tea is emptied into a porcelain or enamel pot, covered with a lid, heated until warm enough to drink and taken on an empty stomach. Three hours after drinking the Super 1 tea, the Super 2 Compound tea is shaken and heated in the same way and immediately taken warm on an empty stomach. The Chinese stress the importance of these directions, stating that it is essential to drink the Super 2 tea *three hours* after drinking the Super 1 tea if results are to be obtained.

It is said that quite often just one treatment consisting of the two-bottle set is sufficient to bring about excellent results. But if the condition does not respond completely to one treatment, the two teas may be taken again the following day, or if necessary for a few days until the desired results are achieved.

According to the Chinese, centuries of experience have proven that the Old-Fashioned Fancy and the Super 1 and 2 Compound Herb teas are harmless.

Further Directions

When heating any of these compound teas, care must be taken that the steamy droplets that form on the inside cover of the pot are not allowed to drop into the tea since this would cause the brew to lose a little of its strength. The Chinese also instruct that for best results when using either the Fancy Compound Tea or the Super 1 and Super 2 set, no fruits or vegetables should be eaten for 48 hours after drinking the tea(s). They explain that the omission of fruits and vegetables from the diet during this 48-hour period allows the herb tea to remain longer in the body, thereby giving it more time to produce its beneficial effects.

Reported Uses

• Mrs. C.S. writes: "I suffered from the miserable condition of cystitis, with a dull ache and straining sensation in the region of the bladder. My urine was a dirty cloudy color with mucus and a strong odor of ammonia. Pills prescribed by my doctor gave only temporary relief.

"Then one day I found out about a Chinese remedy called Super 1 and 2 Old-Fashioned Compound Tea. After taking just two sets of the teas, I found the results were just wonderful. The ache and straining feeling in the bladder were gone, and the urine clear and odorless. There has been no return of the condition in over a year."

• "I was troubled with scalding urine, and backache in the lower part of my body. Sometimes the ache was so intense I could hardly straighten up. My condition was diagnosed as kidney congestion. Since I am a firm believer in natural healing methods, I took the suggestion of a friend who had been cured of a similar problem by using a special Chinese herb tea. It was a formula called Fancy Old-Fashioned Compound tea, and after taking only two bottles, I was completely well again." —Mr. C.R.

•"An X-ray showed that I had small stones in my bladder. At times the pain was very severe. I was terrified at the thought of an operation so on the advice of a Chinese herbalist, I tried a set of Super Old-Fashioned Compound teas. Most happily the pain soon went away and some time later, much to the astonishment of my doctor, there was no longer any trace of the bladder stones!" —Mrs. P.N.

•The following letter was written by a reflex therapist: "There is a Chinese herb formula known as Chinese Super Old-Fashioned Compound Herb tea which seems to have a particular value. I personally know of several people who were troubled with gravel and with stones (kidney, gall bladder, and so on), and they had almost immediate relief after using the Chinese herb compound, with no recurrence of pain or distress. One man was in pain daily and had relief the day he took one set of Super 1 and Super 2 jars of tea. Several months later he said he had no further trouble.

"One interesting thing about this Old-Fashioned Chinese Herb Compound is that it does not have to be used for a long period of time to get results. In every case I know of it has taken only one or two applications of the Super Herb Compound, set 1 and 2 to get results.

"I've never known of any Chinese herb formula for the conditions mentioned that has had such remarkable results so consistently with so many people."

SUMMARY

1. There are a variety of time-tested herbs which are of great value in coping with urinary disorders.

2. In some cases an herb forms a useful remedy when used alone, but is even more effective when combined with other herbs.

3. According to an English herbalist, remarkable permanent cures have been attained with the use of kidney bean pod water for bladder and kidney disorders.

4. It is important to note that results from using the bean pod water could be achieved only with the *freshly made* decoction, and only if taken the same day it was prepared. Even bean water that was more than 24 hours old was found to be of little use.

5. The bean pod water is made from the sliced pods *without the beans.*

6. Anyone deciding to try the bean pod water should start with very small amounts, about a half-glass a day. That amount would not have any therapeutic effect but might indicate if you are subject to any possible adverse effect. Only when you are certain you are not sensitive to the decoction should you attempt using it.

7. Chinese Old-Fashioned Compound Herb Tea is an ancient formula that comes in liquid form and in two strengths: the regular strength called "Fancy," and the stronger strengths called Super 1 and Super 2.

8. The Fancy Old-Fashioned Chinese Herb Tea is also available in powdered form, contained in capsules.

9. The Chinese Old-Fashioned Herb Teas are taken on an empty stomach. Fruits and vegetables should be avoided for 48 hours after drinking the tea(s).

10. If you use the Super 1 and Super 2 bottle set of the Chinese herb compound, it is important that Super 2 be taken three hours after you drink the Super 1.

CHAPTER 6

Herbal Preparations
for the Eyes

Some herbs used for the eyes have an ancient and worldwide reputation. Many of them deal with conjunctivitis, cataract, eye strain, night blindness, and other eye ailments, but patience and perseverance are needed to achieve satisfactory results.

EYEBRIGHT

Botanical Name: *Euphrasia officinalis*
Common Name: Eyebright

Some years ago, a medical doctor residing in Paris became renowned for his successful treatment of certain conditions affecting the eyes. His fame soon spread throughout the city as word got around that many of his patients were able to discard their eyeglasses. The rejected glasses were tossed into an empty tub in the courtyard of his house which gradually become filled as the years passed.

The majority of his patients had their vision affected by some form of eye inflammation; conditions such as blepharitis and conjunctivitis were commonplace. The remedy he prescribed was a simple herb called eyebright (*Euphrasia officinalis*). Generally the herbal preparation was used in the form of an eye lotion; however, in some cases it was also taken internally as a tea made from the dried plant.

Eyebright—a Traditional Remedy

Eyebright is a tiny herb, common in Europe, in northern and western Asia, and in North America. The botanical name *Euphrasia* is taken from the Greek *Euphrosyne*, "gladness," the name of one of the three Graces known for her joy and mirth. It is believed to have been given to the herb because of the effective properties attributed to it as an eye medicine in preserving the eyesight and bringing gladness into the life of the sufferer. It is interesting to note that the French name for this healing plant is *Casse-lunettes* (breaker of spectacles), while the Germans call it *Augentrost* (consolation to the eyes) and the Italians, *Luminella* (light for the eyes).

For centuries eyebright has been regarded as a specific for various diseases of the eyes. It was recommended as an eye medicine by a physician of Mantua who lived about 1329. Herbalists in the 16th century also praised its virtues for treating ailments affecting the sight, and to this day it has retained its popularity among modern herbalists who still recommend its use for the same purposes. In Scotland, the Highlanders prepare an infusion of the herb in milk and anoint inflamed or weak eyes with a feather dipped in it; in Iceland, the expressed juice is used for general ailments of the eyes; in Germany, the herb prepared as an infusion with water is used as an eye bath for tired, inflamed, watering eyes, and for granulated eye lids.

The following information on the use of eyebright is from *Acta Phytotherapeutica*,[1] a Dutch scientific journal on botanical medicine.

> Every student of herbs knows the uses of *Euphrasia officinalis* or eyebright. It is the main herb for protecting and maintaining the health of the eye. It acts as an internal medicine for the constitutional tendency to eye weakness in fluid extract at the dosage of 10 drops three times daily or an infusion of the crude cut herb, one ounce to one pint of water in wineglass doses three times daily.

An even more effective method reported by the journal is a local application of a lotion "made from three drops of fluid

---

[1]Vol. XII, No. 9, 1965, Amsterdam, Netherlands.

extract of *Euphrasia* in an eyebathful of cold water." The eyes are bathed morning and night.

For the treatment of inflammation of the eyelids or the tendency to mucus accumulations in the eyes and redness of the rims of the eye lids, bathing with *Euphrasia* eye lotion should be supplemented by the addition of one drop of fluid extract of *Hydrastis canadensis* [golden seal] in an eye bath of the lotion.

Dr. Jon Evans of England regards eyebright as a highly effective remedy for conjuctivitis which he describes as "a condition exuding white matter which often causes the eyelids to stick together with a smarting and almost unbearable irritation." He recommends an eye bath prepared by pouring one pint of boiling water over one ounce of the herb. The infusion is allowed to stand for one-half hour, then carefully strained through absorbent cotton or a cloth. If the eyes are very painful the lotion should be warmed before using it. The eyes are to be bathed three to four times a day. If the fresh plant tincture is used, only three drops are placed in a tablespoon of boiled water, and allowed to cool before using. A stronger solution may cause the eyes to smart. Whichever method is used, the eyebath should be freshly filled for each eye.

In reference to the value of the eyebright, Swinburne Clymer, M.D., wrote:

EYEBRIGHT

(*Euphrasia officinalis*)

The remedy for sore eyes. An infusion should be made of the leaves and the eyes frequently washed with it. Cold compresses of the same tea should also cover the eyes. It is cleansing and healing to the optic nerve. In conjunction with the external application tea may be made of the root of the plant and taken internally. Half a teaspoonful of the root is sufficient for one tea.[2]

An Impressive Case History of Eyebright Used in Homeopathic Form

A woman had a cyst on the lower right eyelid, as a result of chronic conjunctivitis. Over the years three or four cysts had been surgically removed, and she was fearful of another operation. Both eyes were heavy-looking and inflamed. In addition to

---

[2]*Medicines of Nature* (Quakertown, PA.: Humanitarian Society) 1960.

the cyst the right eye was lumpy, swollen, and "wept" when she was outdoors.

One day someone suggested she visit a homeopathic pharmacy. She took up the suggestion and was given the following prescription: "Euphrasia 6 [eyebright] in tablets, with a recommended dose of two tablets hourly for a day, and then three times daily, and some Euphrasia mother tincture [homeopathic], one drop to be used in an eye bath of water once or twice daily."

Two weeks after she started using the tablets and tinctures, both her eyes were clear and free from inflammation. The swelling of the right eye was entirely gone and the cysts considerably reduced in size.

When the woman went back to her eye specialist he was astonished at her improved condition. He told her he had never heard of Euphrasia but advised her to continue the treatment for another month and return for another examination.

Following her doctor's instructions she bought a month's supply of tablets and tincture. A week later the cyst was barely noticeable, and there was only a very faint trace of inflammation on the eyelids. At the end of the month, she reported that her specialist confirmed undoubted and marked improvement. He advised her to continue with the treatment which was obviously producing such excellent results.

NOTE: In a homeopathic medicine, the number which directly follows the name of the remedy—for example, Euphrasia 6—refers to the rate of trituration. The small white tablets, sweetish in taste, are dissolved slowly under the tongue, never washed down with water or taken at the same time as food.

CINERARIA MARITIMA

Botanical Name: *Cineraria maritima*
Common Name: Dusty Miller

This is a perennial seaside plant which grows along the shores of the Mediterranean. A homeopathic tincture has reportedly produced good results in some cases of cataract. The Dutch Journal, *Acta Phytotherapeutica*, gives the following information.

All opacities of the eye, corneal or vitreous, are best treated with *Cineraria maritima*. The homeopathic tincture of Cineraria is famous as the most effective means of controlling early forms of cataract. One or two drops in each eye morning and nights where there is any sign of trouble is the best safeguard against the development of cataract. Many established early cataracts have been halted and cleared up by the prompt and regular use of Cineraria.[3]

Other qualified sources also report that the most satisfactory results occur when the preparation is used in the early stages of cataract. In these cases, clinical experience and observations have shown definite benefits in halting or even dissolving existing opacities by local applications of this homeopathic herbal remedy.

To obtain more data regarding the effects of *Cineraria maritima* in advanced conditions of cataract, a study was conducted by ophthalmologists. The herbal preparation was employed in 40 cases in which the onset of the disease was over four years; this is past the stage where best results are attainable. Two drops of the liquid were placed in the eyes of each patient morning and night. Results showed that 22.5 percent of the group of 40 patients received beneficial effects.

FENNEL

Botanical Name: *Foeniculum vulgare*
Common Names: Sweet Fennel, Wild Fennel

Fennel has been known since ancient times as a culinary herb and medicine. In Italy the use of the herb dates from the days of the early Romans when gladiators mixed fennel with their food, claiming it gave them strength. Today the plant is still best known to the Italian people, and Italy is its greatest stronghold.

Although a popular culinary herb, fennel has the added distinction of being regarded as a slimming aid and strengthener of the eyes.

A physician to the first Emperor of Germany claimed he saw a monk cured of cataract by his tutor, who applied frequently to the monk's eyes a strong decoction of the whole plant (bruised while fresh, steeped in boiling water, and allowed to cool).

Modern Uses

Fennel is rich in Vitamin A. People lacking in vitamin A not only complain of difficulty in seeing well at night but also

---

[3]Vol. XII, No. 9, 1965, Amsterdam, Netherlands.

find that their eyes are extremely sensitive to light, such as the glare from automobile headlights, TV screens, or the bright reflections from snow.

One woman who drank fennel tea for several months as a reducing aid reported that the tea also produced a favorable effect on her eyes. She writes: "I always drank four cups of tea each day, one before breakfast, one on my coffee break, one before dinner, and one just before going to bed. I did not follow a strict diet but just cut down a little on the starches, sugars, and the fats. Besides losing the extra weight, I received an unexpected health benefit. I had never heard that fennel was good for the eyes, but after only two and a half months of drinking the tea I noticed that an old eye discomfort (bright light pained my eyes) had disappeared."

Fennel seed tea is prepared by placing four tablespoonfuls of the seeds in two pints of boiling water and simmering for five minutes. The covered container is then removed from the burner and allowed to stand for 15 minutes, then strained. One teacupful is taken three or four times daily. It may be reheated if desired.

Eye Bath. A cleansing, strengthening, and refreshing eye bath is prepared with ⅛ ounce each of fennel and eyebright placed in a cup, and boiling water added. The cup is covered with a saucer and the tea allowed to stand until cold. It is then stirred, and strained carefully through absorbent cotton. The eyes are washed with an eyecup every two to three hours, or as necessary.

HONEY

The external application of honey has a great reputation among the ancient Egyptians for producing clearer vision. It was extensively used in inflammation of the eyes and eyelids. The Egyptians also believed that honey dropped into the eyes would cure cataract.

The Germans have always been steadfast believers in the curative power of honey as an eye remedy. For example, during the last century, Fr. Kneipp, renowned priest-herbalist of Germany, wrote: "The purifying and strengthening honey-water for the eyes is well known. Boil a teaspoon of honey in a cup of water for five minutes, and [when cool] it is ready for dipping in the linen for the eyes."

Modern Uses

Natural unheated, unrefined, inorganic honey is a favorite domestic remedy in Germany, France, England, Russia, and elsewhere for treating cataract. One drop of honey is placed into the eye by means of an eyedropper, or the honey may be worked around the edges of the eye with the finger, to bring about penetration. Although any of the different types of honey are used, eucalyptus honey seems to be the most popular.

Honey is also used in many lands as a natural remedy for trachoma (a virus disease of the eyelids). One woman in Canada reported that two of her children contracted the ailment while attending school, as there was an epidemic at the time. When honey was dropped in their eyes with an eyedropper, they were cured in two or three days. By contrast it took three weeks for the other school children to get rid of the same problem. Cataracts were reportedly cured by the same method, i.e., honey dropped into the eyes three times daily.

For twitching of the eyelids two teaspoons of honey are taken at each meal. The condition then generally disappears within a week.

CHINESE HERB COMPOUND

Chinese Old-Fashioned Compounded Herb Tea #3 is a processed herbal formula reputed to be of special benefit to the eyes. One bottle is taken once a month. It is also regarded as a rejuvenation tea. Wrinkles reportedly begin to fade after six months' use of the tea.

Some Interesting Cases

• "The Chinese Old-Fashioned Tea Number 3 is fabulous. It improved my vision almost 100%. It cleared up practically all the spots before my eyes. I could already notice some improvement after taking the first bottle, and have continued using it. I am farsighted, therefore still have to wear my glasses for reading or watching television, but I feel this too will improve with time."
—F.W.

•"One year ago, I had a cataract removed and a permanent lens implanted. My eye did not heal as rapidly it should. It was painful for months. I had to take codeine for the pain. My ophthalmologist told me there was an inflammation and also

muscle contraction. I discussed this with a Chinese herbalist and he gave me a special tea called Chinese Old-Fashioned #3. Within one week the inflammation was gone and the pain greatly reduced."
—M.E.

WITCH HAZEL

Botanical Name: *Hamamelis virginica*
Common Names: Spotted Alder, Snapping Hazelnut, Winterbloom

The generic name, *Hamamelis*, is derived from a Greek word to indicate its resemblance to an apple tree. Early settlers learned of the medicinal value of witch hazel from the native Indians. It was used in Grandmother's day as a household remedy for burns, scalds, and inflammation of the eyelids, and is still in general use today.

Five drops of witch hazel in a eye bath half-filled with warm milk is said to be very refreshing to dull, tired-looking eyes.

Cold packs are also refreshing to the eyes. These are prepared by soaking a large wad of absorbent cotton, or a folded cloth about the size of man's handkerchief, in cold water. Squeeze out, and sprinkle on a little extract of witch hazel. Place over the closed eyes at various moments of the day, for example before getting up in the morning, and when resting after lunch, or during the evening. One pad for each eye may be used. Let them remain for ten minutes or more.

OLIVE OIL

Sometimes foreign particles such as grit, ashes, or dirt accidently get into the eyes. An old-time family doctor book states that two drops of slightly warm olive oil may be dropped directly on the eyeball as a first-aid measure until the services of a physician can be obtained.

In some European countries women apply olive oil to their eye lashes daily, claiming that it makes the lashes grow longer.

CASTOR OIL PLANT

Botanical Name: *Ricinus communis*
Common Names: Castor Oil Bush, Palma Christi

The castor oil plant is native to India, where it is known under several Sanskrit names. It has been cultivated not only through tropical and sub-tropical regions but also in many temperate countries around the world.

Castor oil applied externally is a favorite domestic remedy for coping with sties. Miss. J.E.R. of England writes: "With me, a sty lasts only a few days when anointed with castor oil. A friend of mine had a bad sty. I advised her to use this oil. She did so. She was amazed at its disappearance within two or three days. She passed on this information to another woman whose eyes were troubled in this way, and that lady too was surprised at an almost immediate response. How long will it be before we return to the older and more reliable medicines of proven worth?"

One simple remedy for cataract was suggested by a hospital orderly. It consists of putting one drop of castor oil in each eye once a day for nine days. The treatment is discontinued for ten days, then repeated.

Castor oil applied to the eyelashes and/or the eyebrows at bedtime three times weekly reputedly thickens them and causes them to grow longer.

GOLDEN SEAL

Botanical Name: *Hydrastis canadensis*
Common Name: Yellow Root, Indian Plant, Yellow Puccoon, Eye Balm

Golden seal was used by the Cherokees as a remedy for inflamed eyes, as well as a bitter tonic in stomach and liver disorders.

This plant contains the alkaloids berberine, hydrastine, and canadine. It also contains resin, albumin, sugar, fatty matter, starch, lignin, and a small amount of volatile oil, but the plant owes its virtues almost entirely to hydrastine and berberine.

Many popular preparations for the eyes, such as eye drops, eye washes, etc., included hydrastine as one of the ingredients.

In England, golden seal is used externally as an eye lotion in treating various eye affections, and as a general cleansing application.

The Dutch scientific journal *Acta Phytotherapeutica* states: "Hydrastis [golden seal] tincture of fluid extract applied externally to the cornea in a dilution of two drops in an eye bath will heal a corneal ulcer if used three times daily."[4]

PUMPKIN

Botanical Name: *Cucurbita pepon*
Common Name: Pumpkin

In China the pumpkin is the symbol of fruitfulness and health, and is called the Emperor of the Garden. Pumpkin takes its name from the Greek word *pepon* which means "cooked in the sun." It is a plant of the gourd family, native to India, but is now naturalized and cultivated in almost every country throughout the world.

Pumpkin seeds contain valuable nutritive properties, and many people claim that snacking on the seeds between meals is healthful for the vision. For example, Mrs. D.B. of Wales writes:

"I wonder if other people would be interested to know that I found pumpkin seeds improved my sight. At first when I told my husband this he laughed and said I must be imagining it or it was that my general health had improved. I checked carefully. Always when I couldn't obtain these seeds I had to resort to my glasses. A day came when I heard that the firm concerned was not supplying the seeds anymore and gradually I had to use my glasses more and more. Then I heard that the firm was supplying pumpkin oil capsules. I started taking them and once again my sight improved. Now although I stil have to use my glasses at night for some sewing or reading small print, during the day I can dispense with them, and I am hoping that the improvement will continue until I can leave them off at night also."

SUNFLOWER

Botanical Name: *Helianthus annuus*
Common Name: Sunflower

The botanical name of this plant comes from the Greek words *Helios*, the sun, and *anthos*, a flower. As though magnetized by the run's rays, the disc of the sunflower follows the great solar orb in its course around the heavens. As the sun rises in the morning, the sunflower slowly faces east, then turns

---

[4]Ibid.

upward, keeping face to face with the sun as it climbs higher in the sky. The flower follows the westward direction of the sun in the afternoon, gradually drooping as the sun begins to set. Evening finds the disc of the sunflower completely facing downward. The entire process is again repeated with the rising of the sun on the following morning.

At one time it was thought that the sunflower was native to Peru and Mexico because the Spanish conquerors found it in use there as a sacred and mystic symbol. The Incas worshipped it as a representative of the sun. In the temples, during religious ceremonies, the seeds were eaten, and a large sunflower made of pure gold adorned the breasts of the priestess of the sun. The sunflower is the floral emblem of Peru and the State Flower of Kansas.

In Russia the plant has assumed considerable economic importance. The finest quality of seed is used for food, and regarded as a delicacy by all classes. The oil is considered highly nutritious and is employed for culinary and domestic purposes. In Spain and Portugal the seeds are made into nutritious bread, or roasted like coffee and made into a beverage. The sunflower is considered so useful economically and medicinally that it is one of the regular crops in Germany, Denmark, France, Italy, Japan, Manchuria, Argentina, Egypt, and other lands.

Nutritive Value of Sunflower Seeds

Sunflower seeds contain a marvelous abundance of vitamins and minerals, all the important nutrients that benefit the eyes. The seeds have proved to be effective for treating such conditions as eye strain, intolerance of bright light, farsightedness, blurred vision, eye weakness, and other eye ailments, according to many people who have used them.

• I am 62 years old and have noticed a remarkable strengthening of my eyes since eating sunflower seeds every day."—Mr. J. L.

• "I read somewhere that very few Russian people need to wear eyeglasses because they found sunflower seeds to be powerfully good for the eyesight. So I began eating a couple of small handfuls of the seeds everyday. After about five weeks I found my vision was no longer misty and I could read without my reading glasses."—Mr. R. T.

•"My daughter is a typist and was complaining that the glare from the white typing paper bothered her eyes. I suggested she try sunflower seeds as they helped me so much when I had a somewhat similar problem (I sew a great deal under bright light). She took up my suggestion and has never complained about the glare since."—M. S.

• "Two tablespoons of sunflower seeds eaten daily cleared up my inflamed and sore eyes in four weeks' time. Since I loved the taste of the seeds, I continued eating them every day thereafter. Was I ever surprised and delighted to find later that the frequent quiver and twitching of one of my eyelids, an annoying condition I've had for years, was completely eliminated!"—Miss L. S.

BURDOCK

Botanical Name: *Arctium lappa*
Common Names: Clotburr, Bardana, Personata, Cockle Buttons

Burdock is a coarse biennial ranging from two to three feet in height and bearing purple flowers. It grows freely in waste places and hedgerows.

In herbal medicine, burdock is considered one of the finest blood purifiers. The plant contains a bitter crystalline glucoside, fixed and volatile oils, inulin, vitamin C, iron, niacin, mucilage, sugar, a little resin, and some tannic acid. In Europe the root is used in herbal blood purifying mixtures and pills. The Japanese boil the roots in salted water and eat them with sauce or butter, like salsify. Those living in the rural regions of Russian claim that a broth prepared from burdock roots, when taken daily, alleviates or prevents sties of the eyes, and also stops the hair from falling out.

Drs. Wood and Ruddock recommend drinking a tea made from the seeds or roots of burdock as a highly effective remedy for sties. "A pint of the infusion may be drunk in the course of 24 hours." As a preventative method for those troubled by recurring sties, "Make a strong tea of burdock seeds or ground centaury plant and take a tablespoonful three or four times a day."

The tea is made with one ounce of the seeds or roots to one and a half pints of water boiled down to one point, then strained.

OTHER NATURAL TREATMENTS

Nutrition

Years of research have shown that proper nutrition can have a definite effect on improving vision and in eliminating certain eye problems. According to various authorities, foods rich in vitamins and minerals are essential to eye health. For example, night blindness, from which some ten million Americans suffer, is one of the earliest signs of vitamin A deficiency; cataract patients have been found lacking in vitamin C; calcium is needed for the eye muscles and for the fluid of the eye. The *American Journal of Ophthalmology* suggests that myopia or nearsightedness is due to a deficiency of calcium and vitamin A.

A lack of vitamin B_2 has been found to cause cataracts in both humans and animals. Dr. L. Sydenstricker reported that he successfully treated many cases of opacities with 15 mg of vitamin B_2 daily, plus an adequate diet to patients exhibiting symptoms of vitamin B deficiencies. The opacities were reportedly reversed in nine months.

It has been shown that animals can develop cataract due to a lack of vitamins D, E, pantothenic acid and tryptophane.

Some nutritionists have found that glaucoma patients are usually deficient in vitamins A, B, C, calcium and other minerals. Dr. R. Ulrich forbids his glaucoma patients to drink coffee as he believes there is a connection between coffee and glaucoma.

Dr. Raiford of the Atlantic Eye Clinic of Georgia says the greatest cause of blindness in the United States is clogged-up blood vessels, which he blames in many cases on junk foods. He has achieved some impressive cures by placing patients on a health diet. He also recommends that little or no alcohol be consumed, that smoking should be avoided, and that cooking fat that is solid at room temperature should never be used. He says that vegetable oils should be used instead, but never reheated time and again. He recommends eating fresh fruits, vegetables, and whole grains. According to Dr. Raiford, tranquilizers, birth control pills, and sedatives should be avoided as they can destroy the chemical balance in the body's cells that affect the eyes.

Eye Exercises

A number of eye specialists have recommended certain eye exercises as being helpful for the vision. Following are a few suggestions.

Palming. If you wear glasses, remove them. Sit in a comfortable chair and try to loosen up and relax completely, keeping the mind quiet and at ease. Close your eyes and cover them with the palms of your hands, and without pressure, exclude the light and concentrate on the blackness. Keep the nose free. Be sure your elbows are supported on a table so that you are comfortable. Keep the palms over the closed eyes for about 10 to 20 minutes daily. This practice reputedly helps conditions of astigmatism, squinting, nearsightedness, and eye strain.

Blinking. The healthy eye is always blinking. When you blink, fluid from a small gland is washed down and over the eyeball to keep the eyes moist. The fluid has an antiseptic and cleansing action. Blinking protects the eyes when the weather is windy and dry, and in cold weather it helps to keep the eyes warm. Blinking aids circulation of the lymphatic fluid around the eyes, and the eyes are strengthened by this circulation.

If you become aware that you are staring at a person or object, your attention should be drawn to the fact that you are not blinking. Staring is straining to see, and strain causes imperfect sight. Blink slow and often to "lubricate" the eyes. A few seconds spent on this practice daily can help weakness of the eyesight and help to prevent staring. At any time when reading or sewing turn your eyes away occasionally for a few seconds of blinking.

Sunshine. Sunlight is beneficial to your eyes. Close your eyes and face the sun, and if you wear glasses remove them. Keeping the eyes closed, gently swing the head from side to side, for about ten mintues daily. This practice is considered an excellent method of relaxation to the ophthalmic nerves and muscles. It provides a good supply of blood to the eyes and the lens receives nourishment. After a few days this practice can be followed two or three times daily.

SUMMARY

1. Certain herbs have an ancient and world-wide reputation for dealing effectively with a number of troublesome eye conditions.
2. When using herbs, patience and perseverance are needed to achieve satisfactory results.

3. Teas, eye baths, compresses, eye drops, and homeopathic preparations are some of the ways in which the herbs may be employed.

4. Years of research have shown that proper nutrition and eye exercises help to protect and maintain eye health. They also reportedly strengthen the vision and remedy certain eye ailments.

CHAPTER 7

Nature's Aids for Bowel and Intestinal Ailments

Many people suffer from various bowel or intestinal complaints. Constipation, called "the Great American tragedy," is perhaps the most common health problem of our nation. Along with food wastes, the bowels discharge cellular debris of body tissues, living and dead bacteria, mucus, and so forth. If retained for longer than the normal period in the bowels, this mass of decaying debris offers a breeding ground for many harmful germs. These putrefying wastes cause bowel discomfort, sour stomach, gas, headache, offensive breath, and other distresses associated with constipation. Poisons generated by putrefying wastes become a potential hazard to the linings of the intestines. A feeling of depression and irritability has often been blamed on irregularity.

Kellogg maintained that the problems of constipation and associated autointoxication (a condition resulting from absorption into the blood stream of toxic fecal waste products due to chronic constipation) are the causes of most human ailments. Professor Metchnikoff, a Russian biologist and Nobel prize winner in physiology, concluded that many diseases which affect mankind are caused by toxic types of bacteria which propagate in the large intestine. He was of the opinion that the prevention of such intoxication would not only help man avoid many illnesses, but would also help preserve youth and prolong life beyond the so-called normal span.

Regular daily evacuation of the bowels, then, is an important step in maintaining or rebuilding a clean, pure bloodstream that can keep you feeling healthy and more peaceful.

A Word about the Skin

Somehow the skin is not generally thought of as a vital organ such as the heart, liver, or lungs. Yet one of the most important functions of the skin is that of excretion of waste products from the body. Experiments by noted physiologists such as Lavoiser, Seguin, and others, revealed that the skin eliminates more impurities from the body than do the lungs, bowels, and kidneys combined. A portion of this waste material is discharged through the skin in the form of invisible gases and is called insensible perspiration. This process continues steadily every day and night. Visible perspiration collects on the surface of the skin and is commonly referred to as sweat. Were it not for this system of removing poisonous waste products from the body, the blood would become more and more toxic until it would no longer be able to support life. Therefore this vital function of the skin cannot be stopped or even checked without inviting serious consequences.

An Impressive Case History

Some people do not sweat, even in the hottest weather or when engaged in vigorous exercises or sports activities. In such cases they often experience symptoms of toxemia.

One woman who used a simple natural remedy for eliminating this distressing condition writes: "I wish you would pass this important information along so that others with my problem may be helped also. For most of my life I have suffered from toxemia. It began when I was in my thirties and I noticed a slow decline in my health. I had headaches around my temples and eyes, sometimes slight nausea, and a miserable, sick feeling of being toxic. For years I had a chronic constipation problem, but took care of it with laxatives and enemas.

"I consulted numerous doctors and had many tests and X-rays, but no cause for my toxemia could be found. The symptoms worsened as the years passed, and by the time I was fifty I was not only chronically ill, but was getting desperate as I felt I hadn't long to live.

"One hot summer day while I was resting on the beach, I met an old retired doctor and told him about the terrible toxemia condition I was suffering from. He questioned me for some time, then began to study me closely, looking at my face, arms and hands. 'Have you ever noticed whether or not you perspire in hot weather, or whenever you have been very active?', he asked. I thought about it carefully, and I couldn't recall ever having done so; in fact I had often wondered over the years how I could be dry as a bone even in the hottest weather.

"The good doctor explained that this could be the cause of my toxic condition. He suggested that I put one or two teaspoonfuls of apple cider vinegar in a glass of water and sip one glassful three times daily.

"The first week that I took the vinegar, I noticed a slight film of moisture on my skin, and I was quite thrilled. The second week there was an increase, and by the end of the month I was perspiring normally! The pressures around my eyes gradually left, and so did the headaches and nausea. I was enjoying a marvelous feeling of being healthy and clean inside and out. Life was truly wonderful at long last. I could hardly believe my good fortune at having met such a wonderful doctor. I still take my vinegar water every day, and have learned to adjust the amount. Sometimes I take just one teaspoonful, instead of two, in a glass of water, depending on my needs."

NATURAL REMEDIES FOR BOWEL AND INTESTINAL AILMENTS

Following is a list of remedies for coping with constipation, diarrhea, hemorrhoids, and certain other disorders of the bowels. The list also includes remedies for dealing with various intestinal complaints.

YELLOW DOCK

Botanical Name: *Rumex crispus*
Common Name: Curled Dock

Yellow dock grows in ditches, fields, and meadows, and is very common in Europe, America, China, and other lands. It can easily be recognized by the crisped, curled edges of its long narrow leaves.

Remedial Uses

Yellow dock is classed as alterative, mild laxative, and tonic. It is a favorite domestic remedy for constipation; however it is not considered a laxative in the classical sense, but rather a regulator and normalizer of bowel function.

The tea is prepared with the cut roots. Although hard substances such as roots and barks are boiled continuously for a certain length of time, yellow dock root is an exception and must never be allowed to boil *continuously*. To do so would destroy the active principles contained in the root.

Yellow dock is prepared by placing one teaspoonful of the cut roots in a cup and adding boiling water. The cup is covered with a saucer and allowed to stand for half an hour, then strained. One cup of the tea, reheated, is taken three or four times a day. The tea has a bitter taste which some people enjoy, but for those who do not, it may be sweetened with honey.

Herbalists point out that the problem of constipation varies with different people, so that the amount of yellow dock tea taken daily depends on individual needs. For instance, some may find that an average of three or four cups of the tea daily is sufficient, but others may need to take more, or less.

Case Histories

• "For the past ten years I was troubled with stubborn constipation, and became very irritable at times. I tried many different drug store remedies, but all of them either caused griping pains or loose watery bowel movements, or both. What a blessing it was to finally discover yellow dock root tea. The bowel movements are now perfectly normal, and no griping cramps. I use the tea every day, and don't ever want to be without it."—Mrs. C.C.

• "Please spread the good word about yellow dock tea. My 75-year-old father was bedeviled with chronic constipation. He constantly complained about the laxatives and enemas he was given. One day I went to see an herbalist about the matter. He gave me a bag of yellow dock roots and told me how to make a tea with them.

Two days after starting the tea, my father had a natural bowel movement. It was like a miracle. I give him three, sometimes four, cups of the tea daily, and he has no further trouble with constipation. He no longer needs to take laxatives or enemas. Why isn't this remarkable tea better known to people?"—Mr. J.C.

PILEWORT

Botanical Name: *Ranunculus ficaria*
Common Name: Lesser Celandine

This is one of the earliest of spring flowers, and is distributed throughout Europe, Western Asia, and North Africa. The plant is called Lesser Celandine to distinguish it from the Greater Celandine which belongs to another species. However, it is more commonly known as "pilewort" because of its long-standing reputation as a remedy for piles.

A Word about Piles

The word "piles" is the common name for the medical term *hemorrhoids*. Doctors explain that piles are caused when the upward flow of blood through the rectal membrane is obstructed. Impeding the flow of blood up through the portal vein allows the remaining blood to congest in the veins of the rectum. If the condition continues, the walls of the veins lose their tone and become distended. This distension of blood vessels can be external, often causing the piles to protrude below the rectum. External piles can be seen and felt on the outer rim of the anus, and can range in size from that of a small pea to that of a walnut.

The distension of blood vessels can be internal when the mucous membrane inside the rectum is the only part affected. With internal piles there is invariably a group of veins and arteries involved. The blood vessels are in a varicosed condition and are able to expand or contract according to the amount of blood that is congested in the rectum at any particular time.

If the internal pressure becomes great, the small veins of the rectal membranes can burst, causing a discharge of blood. This discharge relieves the congestion and brings prompt relief to the sufferer, but unfortunately such bleeding can sometimes be so frequent and profuse that the victim develops anemia. Bowel movements may irritate the swollen veins of internal or external piles and also cause them to bleed at times.

In the condition of piles, pain, soreness, itching and burning are often present, especially in advanced cases.

There are many different causes of piles, but the most common source of the trouble is constipation, and severe and repeated straining to move the bowels.

How Pilewort Herb Is Used

Pilewort is classed as an astringent. It is prepared as a tea, one heaping teaspoon of the leaves in a cup, and boiling water added. The tea is allowed to stand for five minutes, then strained. One teacupful is taken cold, three or four times daily.

Pilewort is also used externally in the form of an ointment or fomentations, poultices, or suppositories.

Pilewort is often combined with other herbs for treating external piles. For example, one ounce each of pilewort, cranesbill, yarrow, and mullein are mixed together. One fourth of the mixture is placed in a pint of cold water and brought to a boil. The tea is simmered for five minutes, then strained. One teacupful is taken three or four times daily.

BAYBERRY

Botanical Name: *Myrica cerifera*
Common Names: Wax Myrtle, Candleberry

"This small tree belongs to the family of myrtles. It grows near swamps and marshes, reaches a height of from three to eight feet, and bears globular fruit resembling berries. The berries produce a green wax which burns brightly, and candles made from it are fragrant, and smokeless after snuffing. It has also been used as a sealing wax.

No tree was more honored in ancient Greece than the myrtle, as it was said to belong to the Goddess of Love. The tree also symbolized both the Creation and the preservation of love.

Remedial Uses

Bayberry is classed as astringent, stimulant, alternative, and aromatic. It has a long-standing reputation as a remedy for dysentery. In 1562, Garcia de Ora wrote that the use of the root cured a girl of dysentery when all else had failed. It was also used by the American Indians for the same ailment, as well as for other disorders.

In modern times, herbalists still regard bayberry as an excellent remedy for diarrhea and dysentery. The tea is prepared with one ounce of the cut roots to one and a half pints of boiling water. This is simmered for five minutes, then allowed to stand until cold. One cold cupful of the strained tea is taken two or three times a day. If the tincture is used, one-half to one teaspoon is taken in a small glass of water two or three times a day.

Combined Formula for Spastic Bowel

Bayberry is often combined with other herbs for treating various bowel troubles. Arthur C. Hyde, a medical herbalist of England, cites the following case history of treating spastic bowel, in which bayberry was used as part of the herb formula. He writes:[1]

SPASTIC BOWEL

A middle-aged lady was shown into my consulting room complaining of a condition which had caused her considerable embarrassment for some time. The symptoms were diarrhea alternating spasmodically with normal bowel evacuation, and at the times when the bowel action was looser, there was severe urgency. This was the most trying part of the trouble, especially when she was out shopping or visiting other people. It caused her to lose her confidence and stay at home far too much, and resulted in mild claustrophobia. Her orthodox practitioner had given her a course of medicine which had done no good whatever.

Upon examination of the abdomen I discovered large accumulations of flatulence which led to severe griping pain prior to bowel evacuation. The tissues of the abdomen were slightly distended and tender to touch. The peristaltic wave, moving food material through the digestive system, was very rapid, and this is what aggravated the condition by causing the urgency with which the bowel had to be emptied. The lady complained also of heartburn after nearly every meal, and this reduced her appetite. With lack of sufficient food being taken in, and the excess of liquids and other matter being expelled by the bowel, the patient's weight was dropping rapidly. She was in a state of some tension, and her nervous system was not as relaxed as it should have been. When I commenced the consultation I suspected colitis in some form, but as there was no mucus voided in the bowel motions this additional possibility was ruled out.

The dietary regimen had to be adjusted, as the patient was trying to digest normal foods which were far too coarse and rough

---

[1]*Health from Herbs*, September–October 1969, p. 8.

for a bowel in this nervous state. I advised a diet of bland, smooth foods, such as slippery elm, barley water, oat-flour porridge and fruit juices, while at the same time avoiding meats, pickles and vinegar and, for a time, raw vegetables.

Herbal medicine containing remedies to correct the runaway bowel action, and to balance the stomach acid level, together with the tone of the abdominal nerves, was the answer to the patient's condition. Very soon after commencing to take these remedies regularly, the lady reported a general improvement, not only in the bowel condition, but in her general health too. The feeling of claustrophobia in small rooms rapidly cleared, and her confidence to go out alone built up steadily as the bowel spasms became less severe and less frequent. Her weight increased, slowly for a start, and then more quickly, until she had reached the same weight she used to be before the bowel trouble.

Of course, the progress with herbal medicine is reasonably slow and measured, but this is Nature's way—nothing in a hurry! The "proof of the pudding," so to speak, is in the completely satisfactory way this lady has recovered from her condition. She is now symptom-free, the heartburn having disappeared along with the other nervous troubles, and is able to eat as she wishes. The flatulence in the bowel has also cleared.

The herbal agents used in this case were taken about a quarter-hour before each main mealtime, as this helped to quiet the bowel activity and prepare the stomach to receive food. The remedies also ensured that the whole of the digestive system worked much more efficiently; this is where most of the weight-gain originated, for the patient ate rather less of much lighter foods, but still regained the lost pounds. The prescription included: Roman Camomile, Hops, Catechu, Marshmallow, Prickly Ash, Meadowsweet, Black Horehound, Bayberry.

Should you be a bowel-sufferer like this lady, and wish to treat yourself for it, the following herbs, taken as an infusion or decoction, 15 or 20 minutes before meals, will prove helpful:

Roman Camomile	¼ oz.
Hops	½ oz.
Bayberry	½ oz.
Prickley Ash	¼ oz.
Marshmallow	1 oz.
Meadowsweet	1 oz.

If you are unsuccessful after a short while in correcting this condition of spastic bowel, your best course is to visit your Consulting Medical Herbalist for his advice and help.

AGAR-AGAR

Botanical Name: *Gelidium amansii*
Common Names: Japanese Isinglass, Ceylon Moss

Agar-agar is a brownish-white seaweed collected on the East Indian coast and shipped to other lands. It is a nutritive and demulcent food widely used for aiding regularity of bowel movements in a natural manner, due to its ability to absorb and retain moisture and provide bulk.

Agar-agar can be made into a jelly with one ounce of the powder to 20 ounces of boiling water. It may be flavored with a little lemon or orange juice. Or one teaspoonful of powdered agar-agar can be sprinkled over stewed prunes or other fruit for breakfast.

COLLINSONIA

Botanical Name: *Collinsonia canadensis*
Common Names: Stone Root, Heal All, Knob Root

This is a perennial plant which grows in damp woods from Canada to the Carolinas. The whole plant has a strong odor and a spicy, pungent taste. The name is derived from its discoverer, Peter Collinson.

Remedial Use

The root is the part of the plant used in herbal medicine. Although it has been employed with good effect for a variety of conditions, it is especially valued as an excellent remedy for piles. The root may be prepared as a decoction, or taken in powder form contained in capsules. Herbalists state that two capsules taken twice daily between meals until results are obtained are generally sufficient for most cases. But in more stubborn conditions of piles, the capsules are taken three times daily between meals until definite improvement is noted, then the dosage is reduced to two capsules twice daily.

Collinsonia Tablets and Ointment

Recently an American researcher tested collisonia tablets and a cream for hemorrhoids. The tablets consisted of collinsonia and whey, and the cream is a combination of collinsonia, tea tree oil and golden seal.* Of the 35 hemorrhoid cases studied, most reported prompt relief from pain, swelling, and itching.

A chiropractor on the West Coast reported that he used the tablets and cream, and his hemorrhoid condition was relieved "like magic." He says he also has prescribed them with good effect for his patients.

CARROT

Botanical Name: *Daucus carota*
Common Name: Carrot

Dr. P. Selander of Sweden stated that the use of carrot soup for the treatment of infantile diarrhea has received favorable reports not only in his own country, but also from Belgium, France and Germany.

Dr. Selander describes the method of preparing the soup. One pound of carrots are freshly washed, peeled, and finely chopped, and placed in a pressure cooker with five ounces of water for 15 minutes at 15 pounds. The entire resulting pulp is strained through a fine strainer and diluted with hot sterile water to make one quart. About ¾ of a level tablespoon of salt is added. The carrot soup is generally spoon fed, but may be bottle fed by removing the top of the nipple.

During the first 24 hours of treatment, the carrot soup is usually given at frequent intervals, often every half-hour. In the average child definite improvement should be noted 24 hours after starting the treatment.

An American physician who heard about Dr. Selander's work decided to give the carrot soup treatment a try, since he felt the remedy was harmless and could be started by parents, especially in rural districts where doctors where not available, or at least until their physicians could be contacted. He says that diarrhea (enteritis) should be treated as quickly as possible at its onset, before rapid weight loss takes place.

He reported that he treated over 600 patients in hospitals and in their homes, with carrot soup, without a known mortality. The cases included epidemic diarrhea of a newborn infant, premature infants, infantile diarrhea, diarrhea of older children suffering from acute colitis, and adults with acute enteritis who were truly benefited with the carrot soup treatment.

---

*Both the tablets and the cream are sold in health food stores and herb firms.

The Health Action of Carrot Soup

Carrot soup combats dehydration by supplying water. It replenishes phosphorous, potassium, choline, magnesium, calcium, sulphur, and sodium (especially with the addition of salt), in diarrhea sufferers who have lost large amounts of these important nutrients. Carrots are also very rich in pectin, a known and proven diarrhea remedy. Carrot soup soothes and assists healing by coating the inflamed small bowels, and also has a slowing effect on the growth of undesirable intestinal bacteria. It prevents vomiting by holding the growth of dangerous intestinal bacteria in check, and preventing them from entering into the duodenum and stomach.

GARLIC

Botanical Name: *Allium sativum*
Common Name: Garlic

Garlic, known for many uses, is employed as a remedial agent by herbalists for colitis, dysentery, diarrhea, and other intestinal disorders.

Either the fresh garlic cloves, or garlic in tablet or capsule form (perles) may be used. In persistent cases of diarrhea or dysentery, two tablets are taken four or five times daily; in average cases two tablets three times daily; in mild cases, two tablets once or twice a day. If garlic capsules are preferred, generally one or two capsules are swallowed three times daily, or if needed, four times a day. (Garlic capsules or tablets leave no odor on the breath.)

If a fresh garlic clove is used, it is taken three times a day, between meals. The garlic clove is finely chopped and added to a cup of warm milk or a soup such as clear beef broth. A mouthful of the garlic soup or milk is taken, and at the same time a little of the finely chopped garlic is scooped up from the cup and swallowed with a second mouthful of milk or broth. This is continued until the whole cup of garlic milk or soup has been consumed.

Scientific Studies of Garlic

Medical reports from all parts of the world are confirming the remedial value of garlic for treating bowel and intestinal complaints.

In Germany, Gusganger and Beecher found that garlic was effective against intestinal putrifaction.

Kristine Nolfi, M.D., of Norway, wrote that the use of garlic "kills putrifaction bacteria in the large intestine and neutralizes poisons in the organism itself."

T. D. Yanovich of Russia described his experiments with garlic. He introduced the juice of garlic directly into colonies of bacteria and found that all movement of the bacteria ceased in three minutes. He also added the juice to a culture of bacteria and found that it caused the bacteria to disperse to the edge of the culture. All activity had ceased within the short space of ten minutes.

In Brazil it was reported that the use of garlic cured 300 patients of intestinal infections ranging from enterocolitis to amebic dysentery.

Some Interesting Case Histories

Professor Roos of Germany wrote an article covering his experiences with the use of garlic in treating a variety of intestinal disorders. Following are a few examples of the many remarkable cases histories he cited:

• A woman, 24 years of age, suffered an attack of acute enterocolitis accompanied with nausea, severe body pains, chills and fever, along with diarrhea. She took two grams of garlic three times daily and by the fifth day her condition was normal.

• A doctor became ill with subacute colitis, symptomized by diarrhea and colic pains. He soon became completely well after taking two grams of garlic three times a day.

• For 17 years, a professor had suffered from colitis, dyspepsia, and gas. Sometimes the diarrhea alternated with spells of constipation. He was told to take two grams of a garlic preparation two to three times daily. In two and a half months the patient considered himself cured.

• A doctor, 28 years of age, experienced attacks of diarrhea every time she ate. Her condition became normal after taking two grams of garlic three times daily, for three days.

SLIPPERY ELM

Botanical Name: *Ulmus fulva*
Common Names: Red Elm, Indian Elm, American Elm

Among its many remedial uses, slippery elm is valued for its gentle, soothing action in conditions of colitis (inflammation of the large bowel) and enteritis (inflammation of the intestinal tract). In addition it acts as a buffer against irritation of the mucous membranes and is considered helpful in conditions of dysentery and diarrhea.

The tea is prepared from the powdered bark. Two teaspoons of the powder are placed in a jar, and one-half cup of cold water added. The jar is capped and the mixture thoroughly shaken. It is then poured into a porcelain container and one pint of boiling water and a pinch of golden seal powder are added. The solution is stirred thoroughly until the powders are well mixed and dissolved. One cup of the tea is taken three times daily.

As an accessory treatment, a second batch of the tea is prepared in the same way and used as a bowel injection with a rectal syringe (after the tea has been cooled to lukewarm). If the liquid is too thick to flow freely through the syringe, it may be diluted with a little more water.

Combined Formula

In his medical writings, herbalist Darwent of England covers the condition of colitis. He expresses astonishment at the number of people who suffer from this disorder and says that in his opinion the cause is generally wrong diet, or a number of things such as sudden chilling of the body when heated, impure water, using strong purgatives, drinking ice water—or even worms that sometimes account for the condition. He adds that women of a nervous type are susceptible to colitis. Darwent lists the symptoms and treatment as follows:[2]

Symptoms

Mucous colitis—If the large intestine is affected there is usually dyspepsia, constipation and passing of mucus, skin, or a jelly-like substance from the bowel.

Ulcerative colitis—Diarrhea, sometimes constipation, greenish or yellowish motions, pain of a griping nature; there may be blood, shred or mucus passed in the motions.

The main symptoms in both cases is this passing of mucus or skin by the motions and a feeling of distress and soreness in the abdomen which is aggravated on slight pressure.

---

[2]"A Practitioner's Case Book," *Health from Herbs*, September–October 1967.

Treatment

Never give strong purgatives for constipation. In this trouble, use licorice powder or compound syrup of rhubarb in small doses, frequently if necessary. Give milk only, or slippery elm food till the trouble is well in hand, and revert to solid foods with caution. I have found this formula most successful:

> One ounce marshmallow root
> One-half ounce lady's slippery or valerian root
> One-quarter ounce slippery elm.

Mix well and boil half in two pints of water for 15 minutes. Strain while warm; and the dose is half a teacupful warm, every two hours during the day.

Darwent explains that quick results cannot be expected, adding that it will take perseverance. However he says that he has known the remedy to help restore people to good health who have had colitis for many years.

Diverticulitis

Dr. T.H. Bartram of England advises slippery elm, plus a special diet, for treating the condition of diverticulitis.

Pure slippery elm powder may be taken with hot milk as a beverage once or twice daily. Mix one heaped tablespoonful of the powder to a thick paste at the bottom of the beaker or cup, with a little water. Add, stirring briskly, hot milk, or milk and water, with sweetening if desired. Very soothing and healing. Do not be put off by the taste. Real yummy for those whose taste buds are not their strongest point.

Diet

On Rising: Glass of diluted fruit juice, lemon or rose hip syrup.

Breakfast: A selection from the following: Porridge made from oatmeal. Milk, 8 oz. (preference to goat's milk). Starch-reduced rolls, honey, ¼ oz. butter. Cup of tea, not too strong. Ripe bananas.

11 A.M.: Cup of China or ordinary tea. Agrimony tea or milk, or glass of slippery elm and milk.

Lunch: Salad. Often with the complaint it is not possible to take salad material. However, take as much of mustard greens and water cress as desired, together with baked potato and butter. Any one of the many nutmeat luncheon preparations sold in health stores may be used.

4 P.M.: Cup of tea, Indian or China.

Evening Meal: 8–10 oz. creamed soup made from sieved vegetables and milk. Hot cooked meal, comprising potatoes baked in their jackets. Cooked carrots rubbed through a sieve. No foods from a frying pan should be used. Four ounces puree of sieved vegetables.

Dessert: Milk prepared in any way—junket, custard, yogurt. Jellies. Honey and roll, or cream-cracker and butter. Baked apple. Avocado pear. Dates.

On Retiring: Glass of milk. Slippery elm, or dandelion coffee (dandelion coffee contains no caffeine).

MULLEIN

Botanical Name: *Verbascum thapsus*
Common Names: White Mullein, Torches, Mullein Dock, Velvet Dock

Mullein can be found growing throughout Europe, Asia, and North America. The name is taken from the Latin, meaning "soft," in reference to its large soft leaves. In olden times, flaming torches were made by immersing the spiral flowering stems in molten tallow and letting them dry.

Remedial Uses

Mullein is classed as demulcent, emollient, and astringent. It is considered a bland, nutritious remedy for various respiratory ailments, and for relieving the pain, irritation, and itching of hemorrhoids. An ordinary infusion of one ounce of the leaves to one pint of boiling water is taken frequently in teacupful doses.

As an accessory treatment, poultices or fomentations are prepared from mullein leaves and applied externally, or witch hazel ointment may be used.

Herbalists point out that perseverance is necessary in stubborn cases.

Mullein is also considered valuable for diarrhea, and for strengthening the bowels. In diarrhea, the ordinary infusion is generally given, but if any bleeding of the bowels is also present the tea is prepared with milk. One ounce of the leaves is simmered slowly for ten minutes in a pint and a half of milk, then strained. One cup is taken warm three times daily.

WHEAT BRAN

A daily ration of unprocessed bran in the diet is highly valued as an effective natural means of preventing or relieving constipation. Sufficient fluids such as milk, soup, juice, or broth should always be taken with bran, as bran has the ability to absorb many times its weight in water or watery fluids, and it is the liquid that produces the large, soft stools that pass easily. The bran may be stirred in liquids, or if it is baked into bread or muffins, plenty of fluids should be drunk when the bread or muffins are eaten.

To find the amount best suited to one's own individual needs, it is best to start with one or two teaspoons of bran and gradually adjust the amount until the desired results are obtained, then continue daily with that specific amount.

Note: Herbalists add a word of caution: any food source high in dietary fiber such as bran should not be used for constipation by patients with intestinal stenosis or adhesions.

Scientific Studies on the Value of Bran

In a letter which appeared in a British medical publication, The Lancet, Dr. Harold Dodd wrote: "Constipation is an ailment of so-called civilization and it can be greatly relieved by the way we live. I cannot speak too highly of Surgeon Captain Cleave's prescription—one tablespoonful of unprocessed bran daily. It restores to the diet what the miller has taken out. For several years I have practiced and prescribed a dessertspoon of unprocessed bran and one of unprocessed wheat germ daily. It is moistened according to the taste with milk, gravy, soup, coffee, or fruit juice. In most patients it ensures a daily formed stool as smooth as with liquid paraffin."

In London, Dr. Neil S. Painter and his colleagues reported on a long-term study in which they gave bran to patients with diverticulosis.[3] Seventy patients suffering from diverticulosis were given anywhere from one teaspoonful to nine tablespoonfuls of unprocessed bran daily, each patient adjusting the amount to his or her own personal need. Most of them took their bran with milk, soup, or water, or sprinkled on cereals, the average dose being two teaspoons three times daily. Dr. Painter also placed his patients on a high residue diet, including whole meal bread, vegetables, fruits, and porridge, and advised them to cut down on sugar.

---

[3]"Unprocessed Bran in Treatment of Diverticulosis Disease of the Colon," British Medical Journal, April 15, 1972.

Ninety percent of the 62 patients who continued the program faithfully every day were relieved or completely cured of their symptoms, which ranged from severe colic to nausea, heartburn, tender rectum, constipation, and a bloated feeling. Where previously about 80 percent of the patients had to strain and had stools that were hard and small, their bowels now were regular, their stools were large and soft, and they no longer needed to strain. Patients with the opposite problem were also helped. Prior to using the bran, one individual needed to go to the bathroom six times a day, and another did so twelve times a day. When on the bran diet, each had only two bowel movements daily. Other researchers have reported the same effect, which indicates that bran is a normalizer of bowel elimination.

Another medic, Dr. Marian Troy, adds a warning that if diverticulosis reaches the acute state of diverticulitis, the dietary advice is different, and the old-fashioned program of a low-residue diet applies.

HORSE CHESTNUT

Botanical Name: *Aesculus hippocastanum*
Common Name: Horse Chestnut

This beautiful tree bears pink and white and occasionally yellow flowers. It is grown in towns, gardens, and parks for ornamental purposes. The trees are generally raised from the nuts which are brown, with a very polished and shining skin. The nuts are not edible as human food.

Remedial Uses

In herbal medicine the use of a fresh tincture of horse chestnut is said to relieve the pain of piles and reduce the swelling, and is a very valuable remedy for enlarged vessels and a distended abdomen. It reputedly has a specific action on the capillary circulation of the rectum and on the lower bowel.

Herbalists in Europe have stated they have known of many cases where small doses of the fresh tincture of horse chestnut have cured prolapse of the rectum and colon, and countless cases of piles which have responded to its use.

The fresh tincture is used in the homeopathic form and sold in homeopathic pharmacies. The dose is two to three drops in a little cold water before meals.

Or the homeopathic pills in the 3X potency may be used instead. The dose is four or five of the tiny pills dissolved on the tongue before meals.

SUMMARY

1. Specific herb remedies and natural foods have successfully coped with a variety of bowel and intestinal complaints.
2. The word "piles" is the common name for the medical term hemorrhoids.
3. Piles can be internal or external. They are symptomized by rectal pain, burning, itching, and sometimes bleeding.
4. Nature's aids to help prevent or overcome constipation are not regarded as laxatives, but as normalizers and regulators of bowel functions.
5. When prepared as a tea, yellow dock root must never be allowed to boil *continuously,* for to do so would destroy the root's therapeutic properties.
6. Liquids such as milk, soup, or broth should always be taken when using wheaten bran.

CHAPTER 8

Plant Remedies for Heart and Circulatory Problems

Heart disease is mankind's number one killer. Recently, in one year alone, deaths from heart ailments rose 916,000 in the United States, and over one million in Russia. In Britain, the death rate from this disease in ratio to the population is the highest in the world.

Although there are many different types of heart trouble, one of the most common is palpitation or tachycardia, which affects nearly everyone at some time or other, to a greater or lesser degree. In this condition, the trouble occurs in spasms, and the heart beats very rapidly, the frequency reaching 170 beats or more per minute. The heart beat may be even or irregular.

There are many different causes of palpitation. In some cases it may occur after a heavy meal, especially if the person is troubled with indigestion. In this case, there may be a sense of uneasiness around the heart, difficulty in breathing, flushes of heat or chilliness, headaches, apprehension or anxiety, and sometimes faintness.

There are other causes that interfere with the action of the heart such as tight clothing, anemia, bronchitis, asthma, or flatulence, and palpitation is often a symptom in women during the menopause. Constipation, alcohol, smoking, and drinking strong coffee can also bring on an attack. Some people become highly excitable or nervous when entering unfamiliar places, or waiting in reception rooms of dentists or doctors, and this in turn may cause heart palpitations. When the system is toned up and strengthened, the nerves are not as easily excited. Tachycardia may also occur after an illness, due to weakness, if the patient resumes his normal duties before he has regained his strength.

Palpitation can often be traced to a reflex disturbance originating from such organs as the liver, kidneys, or stomach. However, it may be a symptom of heart trouble, and sometimes it is the only symptom of early disease of the heart, so it is always wise to obtain professional advice.

Presented here are some of the natural aids used in various parts of the world for treating heart and circulatory disorders.

HAWTHORN

Botanical Name: *Crataegus oxycantha*
Common Names: Crataegus, English Hawthorn, May Bush, Haw, Mayblossom.

This small thorny tree or shrub is native to Europe, Africa, and Asia, but is naturalized in many areas of North America. It bears crimson flowers and produces red fruit (hawthorn berries). Its generic name, *Crataegus oxycantha*, is derived from the Greek words *Kratos* (hard, in reference to the hardness of the wood), *oxus* (sharp), and *akantha* (a thorn).

Remedial Uses

During the last century it was learned that Dr. Greene, an Irish physician of Ennis, County Clare, Ireland, was achieving amazing results with the use of a secret remedy for treating heart disorders. People came from many parts of the world to be treated by him, and he aroused the jealousy of the medical profession by his great success. On his death in 1894, his daughter revealed that the remedy he had been using was a tincture of the ripe berries of the English hawthorn. By 1898 many doctors and herbalists began administering the tincture to their heart patients with remarkably good effects.

As a result, there exists a great deal of clinical data published early in the century, which demonstrates the effectiveness of hawthorn berry in coping with various heart ailments. As space will not permit quoting from all these publications, a few examples are cited as follows:

In the *Homeopathic Recorder* of May 1908, Dr. Crawford R. Green stated:

The action of Crataegus is so broad that there are few heart conditions it does not include, and none that counterindicate it. In fact, it may be regarded as approaching a specific for cardiac conditions in general. It acts both as a powerful heart tonic and as a stimulant. It profoundly affects the circulation, strengthening the weak pulse and regulating its rhythm, correcting alike tachycardia [rapid heart beat], brachycardia [very slow heart beat], or simple arrhythmia, apparently regardless of cause.

Its action in valvular heart conditions is truly remarkable, whether the mitral or aortic area be affected. It seems to have positive power to dissolve valvular growths of calcareous or vegetative origin. It is of value, too, in heart conditions caused by, or associated with, anemia.

Crataegus has saved many lives in cases of organic disease with failing compensation. In the pronounced edema of such conditions, it manifests a diuretic action in every respect rivaling that of Digitalis, Apocynum and Strophanthus. Some observers have found the extreme dyspnea frequently associated with these conditions to be a leading indication for its employment. Unquestionably, it has a powerful action upon the pneumogastric nerve, correcting its inhibitory function when heart failure is imminent as a result of over-stimulation.

In heart pains of various kinds, where we so frequently think of Cactus, Spigelia, Kalmia, and their allies, Crataegus often gives relief when other remedies fail. In angina pectoris it is of indubitable value. Jennings has reported its use in a series of forty cases of true angina with remarkably good results.

As a heart stimulant and sustainer in the infectious fever, Crataegus is of the greatest service. In diphtheria, typhoid, pneumonia and all other toxemic conditions, it may be confidently prescribed as a routine measure upon the least sign of a flagging heart. In such conditions, it gives results far safer and more effective than alcohol, Digitalis or Strychnia. When employed in this manner, I have frequently seen lives saved with it when I am confident that any other form of stimulation would have failed. In two cases of typhoid fever I have seen heart murmurs disappear within twenty-four hours after its administration, reappear within a few hours when the remedy was experimentally discontinued, and again disappear upon its readministration.

In fatty degeneration of the heart, where, above all, we must guard against the dangers of over-stimulation, Crataegus is an absolutely safe remedy. For this reason, pulmonary tuberculosis, so generally associated with fatty heart, presents a field of exceptional utility. In the tubercular wards, it has been shown that Crataegus will often tide a patient over critical periods when adrenalin is of the transient action, and Strychnia, always dangerous in pulmonary tuberculosis, would expand the heart and as surely kill the patient.

In shock, in collapse, in syncope of cardiac origin, Crataegus gives excellent results when administered alone or in conjunction with any other stimulant that seems immediately indicated.

A summary of the symptoms for which Crataegus has been administered would be an epitome of the symptomology of heart disease in general. Feeble and irregular pulse; valvular murmurs; edema; dyspnea; pallor; cutaneous chilliness; blueness of fingers and toes; circulatory disturbance; heart inflammations; heart pain—all these symptoms and many more are attributed to it by various observers.

The dosage of Crataegus is usually given as five to fifteen drops of the mother tincture [homeopathic], repeated every six hours. As the remedy has no cumulative action, it may be repeated at more frequent intervals in severe cases with perfect impunity. As a heart tonic and sustainer the administration of seven to ten drops, three times a day to adults, or two to four drops to children, gives excellent results. Clarke recommends it during or immediately after a meal, as otherwise it may cause nausea. I have, however, repeatedly given it upon an empty stomach, and in only one instance have observed it to cause gastric disturbance. . . . The preparation used is of importance, for the tincture should be prepared from the ripe hawthorn berry and not from the whole plant.

Here are a few excerpts from an article by J. A. Hofheimer, M.D., published in *American Medicine* for September, 1916:

Crataegus is essentially a mild cardiac tonic. It is perfectly safe and has no poisonous effect. It can do no harm in aortic disease, and it is worthy of a trial in these troublesome cases. In fatty degenerations and in heart lesions associated with the high arterial pressure it should be a useful agent.

Fyfe's (Eclectic) *Materia Medica* mentions the indications for giving Crataegus to be "cardiac neuralgia; palpitation; intermittent pulse with increased rate; extreme dyspnea on slight exertion, usually accompanied with pain in the cardiac region; valvular deficiency, with or without enlargement. Crataegus is a remedy of great power in both functional and organic wrongs of the heart. In angina pectoris and in valvular deficiencies most wonderful results have been obtained from its exhibition after the failure of some of the best known heart remedies."

Dr. Hofheimer adds that he himself has also had considerable experience with the use of Crataegus and has prescribed the tincture in several cases "always with good results." Following are two examples of the cases he cites:

William G., Jr., age 18, had recently been refused a policy in a well-known life insurance company, on account of "cardiorenal disease," albumin having been found in his urine. He is a robust-appearing young man five feet eight inches tall, and weighs 163 pounds. He has never had any serious illness, and his family history is excellent.

Examination of the heart reveals cardiac dilatation with a faint mitral systolic murmur, due to insufficiency. Blood pressure 135 mm., and the pulse 96. He admits that he frequently has noticed palpitation and slight precordial pain, especially after walking quickly. Several urinalyses have been made, showing uniformly high specific gravity (ranging from 1025 to 1040); increased acidity, and albumin present in a few specimens, especially in the evening urine, and only after partaking of a meal of high protein content, containing meat or eggs. No casts nor sugar found at any examination.

February 13, gave alkaline diuretics and specific tincture of Crataegus in ten-drop doses three times daily. March 5, slight improvement in cardiac action. No albumin. March 19, continued improvement. Now taking only Crataegus in fifteen-drop doses twice daily. April 16, has been reexamined by insurance company's doctors and has been issued a policy. July 9, he has been steadily taking Crataegus twice daily since last note. Examination today shows a heart regular in action, without murmur; pulse, sitting 75; after hopping, 90. No distress over cardiac region; blood pressure, 130, and urine free of albumin.

Mrs. J., age 57, has had frequent mild anginoid attacks for more than a year. Examination shows an intermittent pulse at irregular intervals; rough systolic mitral murmur; blood pressure 175 mm., systole, and pulse 78–90. After taking Crataegus a few weeks the angina disappeared, and the pulse became more steady and regular. Her son, a physician, reports that she continues to improve, and is only taking the Crataegus; also that while formerly there was a slight albuminaria, this has now disappeared.

Modern Uses

Hawthorn has come under modern scientific investigation. Ullsperger (*Pharmazie*, 1951, 141) isolated a yellow substance from English hawthorn and found that it produced dilation of the coronary vessels. It was reported by Faschauer (Deutche med. Wchnschr., 1951, 76, 211) that 100 heart patients requiring continuous therapy were given the liquid extract of hawthorn and the results were generally beneficial. Marked subjective improvement was noted in patients with mitral stenosis and patients with heart disease of old age. In other patients, digitalis could be either temporarily discontinued or considerably reduced when hawthorn extract was administered.

Medical herbalists of Europe and elsewhere still regard the fluid extract or tincture of hawthorn as a fine heart tonic. For example, Dr. W. Smith of England writes:

> The fruit or berry [hawthorn] is the part principally used in botanic medicine. Where the pulse is rapid and feeble it seems of particular value because of its tonic action on the heart. In valvular insufficiency, dyspnoea (difficult breathing) and in hypertrophy (enlargement) it is also of great value.
>
> It has proved successful in many cases of so-called heart failure, and also in Angina Pectoris. Small doses often seem to have a better effect than the usual large doses often prescribed. The fluid extract should be given in doses of from 10 to 30 drops, three or four times daily.
>
> In practice I have prepared a tablet from the dried, powdered berries, and prescribed them in doses of one or two tablets three times daily with very good results.

Dr. T. H. Bartram refers to the value of hawthorn as follows:

> A well-known herbal sheet-anchor for general heart trouble is, of course, hawthorn. Berries can be used with success in most cardiac disorders, especially hypertrophy. It is appropriate where the psychological pattern is one of melancholy and irritability. It works best where the pulse is weak and rapid, with concurrent dropsy and dyspnea (labored and difficult breathing). It is doubtful whether digitalis, the most widely used heart remedy in the world today, can accomplish more than this common tree. One thing is certain—the menacing cumulative effects of digitalis are avoided in treatment by hawthorn.

In reference to hawthorn berry, Dr. Eric Powell writes:

> This is prepared in tincture or fluid extract form and the dose varies from fifteen to sixty drops in water before meals three times daily, young people requiring smaller doses than adults. Crataegus is probably the best rejuvenator of the heart ever discovered, and it is absolutely harmless. The herbal schools have employed it with great success since the discovery was made known. Home-

opaths are also enthusiastic about the results achieved. Although it may be given in homeopathic potency, it is usually administered in the form of the tincture or fluid extract. Valvular deficiency, enlargement, and some forms of inflammation yield to the gentle influence of Crataegus.

The writer is quite satisfied that it is without equal as a remedy for most heart cases, and he speaks with some authority as he himself was cured with Crataegus when given up to die of heart disease when a child. He has been using Crataegus professionally for some thirty-five years with the most pleasing results.

Dr. Powell gives additional advice for heart conditions:

Foods which have a strengthening effect on the heart are asparagus, apples, honey, parsley and whole grain (the germ of wheat is rich in vitamin E which is definitely a strengthener of the heart). Fresh lemon, sweetened with honey, is probably the best beverage for all heart cases for it not only tones the heart valves and muscles but improves the circulation. There is reason to suppose that quite a number of suspected heart disease cases have nothing to do with the organ itself, but are forms of indigestion causing distension which presses on the heart and produces heart symptoms. Hence the cure lies in correcting the digestive function.

All sufferers from heart trouble should give the feet—only the feet—a hot bath every night before retiring. Have the water well up over the ankles and as hot as possible, adding more hot water every minute or so. Bathe the feet for about ten minutes; well dry, then pull the toes and loosen up the feet with the hands. This will help to equalize circulation, soothe the nerves, remove congestion around the heart and induce restful sleep.

BUCKWHEAT

Botanical Name: *Fagopyrum esculentum*
Common Name: Buckwheat

The use of buckwheat in cases of high blood pressure, and as a tonic and blood purifier, has been known to herbalists for many years. From this plant, science has extracted precious rutin, the wonderful strengthener of the capillaries, and this valuable substance is available in tablet form as a dietary supplement.

The Health Value of Rutin

Your blood capillaries are a natural barometer of health and energy. High blood pressure often accompanies advancing years;

when it is present in conjunction with fragile capillaries, a dangerous condition is created. The increased pressure may burst the ends of the capillaries causing either internal hemorrhage, retinal hemorrhage (blindness) or cerebral hemorrhage (stroke).

Rutin is considered a good remedy for high blood pressure, and a protection against increased capillary fragility and permeability. Dr. Hollenstein and his colleague experimented with lab animals by increasing their blood pressure high enough to cause hemorrhaging of the small blood vessels. They gave rutin to one group of animals ten days before they induced high blood pressure. Only those animals that were given rutin showed no evidence of hemorrhaging.

Some cases of angina have been helped with the use of rutin. Mr. B. T. of England writes: "Thirteen years ago I was knocked over with angina. For five and a half years I was bedbound as well as house-bound. Then I started taking rutin, being told that in three weeks I would experience improvement.

"I did. Now I can walk a little and work a little without 'blacking out' as I did frequently. I still take some every day. Over the past seven and a half years I have, in odd half-hours of work, made a host of hand-crafted articles for my friends and myself, and hope to continue to do so.

"I hope this will be of interest to other sufferers of angina. My condition was diagnosed 'angina on effort.' It still leaves me with a shaky hand, as my writing shows."

MULBERRY

Botanical Name: *Morus alba*
Common Name: Mulberry Tree

The mulberry is a handsome tree with a picturesque appearance. It does not bud until after the frosts are over, and for this reason it has been called "the wisest of trees." The same idea is indicated in its generic name *Morus* which is derived from the Latin word *mora*, meaning "delay," in reference to the late budding of the tree.

The cultivation of the mulberry tree in Asia dates from antiquity, and several varieties are found in all parts of China. The fruits of the common mulberry are known in Chinese as *Shen*. When fully ripened they are called *Hsun* or *T'an*. In commerce they are sold under the name of *Sang-shen-tzu* and made into a jam called *Sang-shen-kao,* in which form the fruits are preserved for medicinal purposes.

The tree has now been cultivated in other parts of the world.

Remedial Uses

Mulberry juice from the ripe berries, diluted with water and taken in considerable quantities, is reputed to improve the circulation and to produce a tonic effect on the heart. It is also said to induce diuresis and therefore to be helpful in some cases for relieving conditions of cardiac dropsy.

A Scientific Study

According to a medical study, 18 heart patients were treated by mulberry therapy, and all but two showed marked improvement. Pain and shortness of breath were reduced and in some cases swelling of the ankles disappeared.

GARLIC

Botanical Name: *Allium sativum*
Common Name: Garlic

Garlic has a long-standing reputation as a natural remedy for reducing high blood pressure. A fresh clove may be finely chopped and added liberally to foods, or the perles which consist of garlic oil may be substituted. The perles provide the same benefit of garlic nutrients, but leave no odor on the breath since they do not dissolve until reaching the lower digestive tract.

Generally, one to three garlic perles are swallowed with a small glass of water three times a day.

Scientific Studies of Garlic

French scientists Poullard, Aguli, Noether, and Leo reported that garlic reduces high blood pressure.

Ortner in Germany cited consistent reduction of high blood pressure in cases treated with garlic. Other scientists in Germany reported that in treating human hypertension, garlic helped 19 out of 20 cases tested in advanced arterial disease.

Kristine Nolfi, M.D., of Denmark, considers garlic to be a normalizer of the blood pressure. In her medical opinion it "lowers too high blood pressure and raises one which is too low."

(This action reportedly does not interfere with normal blood pressure.)

According to Fischer, giddiness and oppression of the head with noises in the ears, especially that form accompanying arteriosclerosis with feelings of anxiety, find a nearly specific remedy in garlic.

Scientists in England reported 25 uniformly successful experiments in relieving hypertension with garlic.

Dr. Piotrowski of the University of Geneva reported on the use of garlic in treating about 100 patients with high blood pressure. In 40% of the cases, the treatment produced a drop of at least two centimeters in blood pressure. Subjective symptoms such as dizziness, back pains, headache, angina-like pains, and difficulty in concentrating began to vanish within three to five days after the administration of garlic was started. In treating his patients, Dr. Piotrowski explained that he began by administering fairly large doses, which were gradually diminished over a period of three weeks. The smaller doses were then continued for the balance of the treatment.

Dr. Piotrowski also mentioned that the expected drop of two centimeters in blood pressure generally takes place after about a week of garlic treatment. He recommends that many more doctors include garlic therapy in treating hypertensive patients.

Literally scores of other scientific research findings from all parts of the world parallel and confirm the reports cited above.

Garlic and Heart Attacks

Professor Hans Reuter found that the use of garlic reduces the danger of heart attacks in people who eat rich foods, as it helps clear the fat accumulating in their blood vessels.

In an important experiment, volunteers were fed butter and given 50 grams of garlic oil in gelatin capsules. It was found that their cholesterol level was considerably lower than that of a group fed butter without garlic. In another test, patients ate three grams of fresh garlic daily, and after one month their cholesterol level had dropped markedly.

According to Professor Reuter, garlic provides an added bonus. Not only does it drive out unwanted fats from the blood, but further tests revealed that in some cases it is more effective than penicillin and other antibiotics.

In India, Drs. Bordia and Bansal of the Department of Medicine, R.N.T. Medical College, Urdapur, conducted studies of the use of garlic supplements on ten healthy volunteers. In these subjects, the average level of serum cholesterol was found to be 221. They were then fed a diet high in fats and in just three hours their serum cholesterol rapidly rose to 237. However, when these subjects were given a fatty diet with garlic supplementation, their average cholesterol serum of 229 decreased to 213 after three hours. In addition, their blood coagulation time became longer. This is important since many Westerners have a slight tendency to form blood clots too fast.

The doctors concluded that for patients inclined toward cardio-vascular disease, garlic could be recommended for long-term use without danger of toxicity

ONION

Botanical Name: *Allium cepa*
Common Name: Onion

The medical profession in Europe has taken much interest in the therapeutic possibilities of onions for treating high blood pressure and other problems of the circulatory system. For example, a team of British doctors has demonstrated with tests on humans that onions fried or boiled can help increase the blood's capacity to prevent or dissolve deadly internal clots. In the tests, convalescent patients were given a portion of onions along with their breakfast or lunch.

Medical research in the United States has shown that raw onions contain about a quarter milligram of prostaglandin in each bulb. Prostaglandin is a hormone that is well known for lowering high blood pressure. (Since onions and garlic are quite similar, it is believed that garlic may also contain prostaglandin.)

Because of the strong diuretic action that onions produce, French doctors have employed them as a three-day treatment for the elimination of fluid in the cardiac and pleural sacs.

VEGETABLE OILS

Through extensive research, American, British, Russian, and other medical teams have agreed that a prime factor in preventing atherosclerosis (a type of arteriosclerosis or hardening of the arteries) is a cholesterol-lowering diet. They also believe that atherosclerosis is chiefly responsible for the steadily growing menace of coronary thrombosis. The findings of these countries show that increased substitution of vegetable oils for animal fats in the diet is one of the best methods of reducing the cholesterol level in the blood.

Dr. Hugh M. Sinclair, Fellow of the Magdalen College, and for many years Reader in Human Nutrition at the University of Oxford, has contributed an important part in the recent conclusions of modern heart specialists. In his own research he has repeatedly found that the substitution in the diet of corn and other vegetable oils for animal fats has a pronounced and undeniable cholesterol-lowering effect.

Dr. Sinclair says:

> Processing and sophistication of foods have destroyed the unstable helpful fats we need which are present in such natural oils as unhydrogenated corn oil, and have created stable harmful fats. The harmful saturated fats are, as the American Heart Association reported recently, present in considerable amounts in most cooking fats and margarines. The helpful highly unsaturated fats occur in vegetable seed oils such as corn oil, cotton seed oil and soybean oil.

Dr. V. Socolovsky gave a report at the Third Annual Congress of Dietetics, held at Church House, Westminster. He revealed that over 500 Russians with coronary atherosclerosis had been subject to laboratory tests. The results enabled Dr. Socolovsky and his colleagues at the Academy of Medical Science for the U.S.S.R., Moscow, to recommend a diet in which one- third of the fats are oils having a high unsaturated fatty acid content for the treatment and prevention of coronary atherosclerosis. Dr. Socolovsky reports that "of the tested oils, corn and sunflower oils have cholesterol-lowering activity."

Mrs. Dorothy Revell, an American dietician, wrote:

> An important principle involved in a cholesterol-lowering diet is the ratio between unsaturated and saturated fats in the daily intake. For every gram of saturated fat there should be two or three grams of unsaturated fat.
>
> Frequently when there is a high level of cholesterol in the blood there is a deficiency of a fatty acid called linoleic acid, which must be supplied in the body from the outside to act as a transportation agent in carrying the cholesterol along the blood stream.
>
> Because of a high linoleic acid content and the fact that it is easily obtainable, corn oil is the preferred unsaturated fat. In my area, Mazola corn oil is readily available and economic to use for all forms of cooking—browning meat, grilling fish, baking cakes and cookies. For some of my patients, I recommend an ounce of

corn oil to be taken first thing each morning as a good start to the day.

Dr. Bartram points out that control of cholesterol is important with regard to the condition of noises or ringing in the ears:

Roaring in the ears [tinnitis] may be due to a number of causes, including high blood pressure, kidney trouble, or heart problems. In dealing with tinnitis, the control of cholesterol is important. Unsaturated fats such as corn oil and sunflower oil have earned popularity because of their low cholesterol potential. Vitamin E is wonderfully sustaining to the cardio-vascular system and assists vitamin C in maintaining resilience of the veins and arteries. Both are helpful for tinnitis.

Studies in France subsidized by the Institut d'Hygiene indicates that the use of olive oil can effectively reduce blood cholesterol. For approximately four months a number of hospital patients suffering from high blood cholesterol were given as much olive oil to drink as they wanted, but no other oil or fat was allowed. At the end of that time, the cholesterol level of seven patients dropped 26 percent. In ten others, it dropped 14.2 percent. It was stated that it is well known that Mediterranean peoples who are great consumers of olive oil "are generally less affected with atheromatoses (arteriosclerosis or hardening of the arteries) than the Anglo-Saxon."

In Zagreb, Yugoslavia, two groups of people were experimentally observed. One group was given olive oil while the other consumed animal fats. The group using animal fats had about 20 percent more cholesterol than the group using olive oil.

TIENCHI GINSENG

Botanical Name: *Panax notoginseng*
Common Names: Tienchi, Sanchi

Ginseng is one of the most highly prized botanicals in the Chinese materia medica. There are several varieties, one of which is called *tienchi*, or *sanchi*. The root, which is valued for its medicinal properties, contains saponins, flavonoids, and sterols which produce a beneficial action on the circulatory system, especially for problems of the veins and arteries.

Tests at the Beijing Institute of Physical Culture showed that the use of tienchi strengthened the constitution, improved the functioning of the cardiovascular system, and helped the body return to normal after exercising. Climbers at 15,000 feet on the Tibetan plateau, who had taken tienchi, had no trouble with irregular heart beat, whereas others who did not take tienchi had irregular changes in their electrocardiagrams.

A clinical preparation of tienchi was given for two months to 680 hospital patients suffering from coronary disease and angina pectoris. The therapeutic rate effect was 60–95 percent and electrocardiagraph improvements were 40–50 percent. It was found that powdered tienchi can reduce the number of attacks of angina pectoris, and quickly eliminate or alleviate the symptoms. Patients who depended on nitroglycerine in tablets were able to reduce the dosage.

When tienchi is taken regularly, cholesterol and lipid metabolism seem to improve, which lessens hardening of the arteries and several other problems of older people.

Another Form of Ginseng

There is a product on the market called Compounded Super Ginseng Roots Tea. It is prepared from 16 selected roots, consisting of the main principal ginseng root and 15 assistant and related varieties of ginseng roots. This Chinese processed herbal compound comes in the form of hard, compressed nuggets (about the size and shape of marshmallows). A tea is made by placing one of the nuggets in a cup and adding boiling water. The nugget quickly dissolves as the tea is stirred. (This product is also available in capsules.)

Therapeutic Action

Each of the 16 roots in the Chinese herbs formula was reportedly selected for its therapeutic and tonic action on a specific part or parts of the body. For example, the principal ginseng root is for the heart and sex glands, three assistant roots are said to support the bone structure, bone marrow, ligaments, and cartilage; another root is for the stomach and digestion; one is for the eyes; another for the nerves, and so on.

As well as for many other uses, this herbal compound is valued by the Chinese for its reputed ability to normalize high blood pressure. One cup of the tea is taken three or four times daily, for approximately six or seven weeks. Mild cases generally take a shorter period of time, and very severe cases may take somewhat longer.

Some Interesting Cases

• One man wrote: "About five years ago I suffered from high blood pressure. Then at a friend's suggestion, I began to drink Compounded Super Ginseng Roots Tea. In the next thirty days my blood pressure gradually returned to normal and has remained within normal limits since then."

• Mrs. W. reports the following: "There are no words to express my feelings adequately for all the benefits I have received from using Chinese Ginseng Roots Compound Tea. Two years ago I was in very poor health, with extremely high blood pressure, and I also suffered from indigestion, restless sleep, and various aches and pains somewhat like rheumatism.

"A Chinese herbalist advised me to take the Ginseng Roots Compound. It was the best advice anyone has ever given me. Within a few days of drinking the tea, I began to feel better. As the weeks passed and I continued drinking the tea daily, the improvement was remarkable. Now after two months, my blood pressure is normal. I sleep fine, the aches and pains have disappeared, and I no longer suffer from indigestion. I feel just wonderful."

• Mrs. Y., a woman in her late sixties, was troubled with high blood pressure, and also complained of heart pains whenever she exerted herself. She reports that taking the Ginseng Roots Compound Tea every day for several weeks normalized her blood pressure and eliminated the heart pains.

• Mr. S. suffered from high blood pressure and gout. He says that both conditions have greatly improved as a result of drinking the Chinese Ginseng Roots Tea.

GINGER

Botanical Name: *Zingiber officinalis*
Common Name: Jamaica Ginger

Ginger is a perennial herb native to Asia. It is produced commercially in many countries, but the best is reputed to be that grown in Jamaica.

Ginger is used in Chinese medicine and is also a favorite ingredient in Chinese cooking.

According to news reports, it is the opinion of researchers at Cornell University Medical College that ginger may help prevent strokes and hardening of the arteries. During tests on agents to slow down blood clotting, a lab technician who was checking blood cells or platelets that he had donated for the study noticed they weren't clotting as they should. He recalled that the night before, he had eaten a considerable amount of ginger marmalade, and further, that studies at the University of Minnesota had linked similar antiplatelet activity to Chinese food. The technician then dropped an extract of ginger on normal platelets and found that they too failed to clot.

A hematology researcher says it is believed that a substance in ginger called *gingerol* inhibits an enzyme that causes cells to clot. The same enzyme is blocked by aspirin, proven effective in preventing recurrence of so-called "little strokes." These attacks are triggered by microscopic artery clots which flow through the bloodstream until they block arteries in the brain.

MOTHERWORT

Botanical Name: : *Leonurus cardiaca*
Common Names: Lion's Tail, Lion's Ear, Herb of Life

This perennial plant has been naturalized from Europe and Asia. It ranges from two to five feet in height and is found growing in fields, pastures, banks, and roadsides.

The Health Value of Motherwort

Motherwort has been valued for centuries as a heart tonic, and it is for this reason that the herb was given the botanical name of *cardiaca*. The plant contains an abundance of calcium chloride. Scientists have found that this mineral compound is necessary for the health of the muscles. Since the heart is a muscle, it requires calcium for strength and to regulate the rhythm of the heart beat. The body also requires calcium for controlling the electric impulses that are transmitted through the nerves.

Szekely writes: "Calcium is the dominant nerve controller and powerfully affects the cell formation of all living things and regulates nerve action. It governs contractability of muscles and rhythmic beat of the heart."

Remedial uses of Motherwort

Motherwort has retained its age-old reputation as a remedy for weakness of the heart, heart palpitations, and poor circulation.

It is also considered valuable for female disorders and reputedly has a very good effect on the womb.

Medical Herbalist Newman Turner of England cites the following use of motherwort:

Motherwort is an old remedy for simple heart conditions, providing a mild tonic and an effective preventative of heart disease. it is a gentle antispasmodic, beneficial in patients who become nervously aware of the heart and concerned about their hearts, possibly through nervous reflex. It is especially useful in heart conditions, the menopause, and menstrual abnormalities.

Up to one-half or even one dram of fluid extract of Leonurus [motherwort] may be taken. This is the main ingredient of a famous old heart pill still sold by leading herbal wholesalers.

Dr. Jon Evans suggests the following method of using motherwort:

As to preparation, an infusion can be made from the herb. One ounce to one pint of boiling water, to be taken in wineglassful doses three times a day after meals. If the preparation is taken in the form of a fluid extract the dose is ½ to 1 drachm. [One-half to one teaspoonful in a small glass of water.]

Motherwort is also used for the relief of leg and foot cramps. It is prepared as a tea, one pint of boiling water poured over one ounce of the herb. After steeping for ten minutes, it is strained, and one teacupful is taken four times daily.

CRUDE BLACKSTRAP MOLASSES

Blackstrap molasses is very high in minerals, and contains most of the valuable B complex vitamins. A deficiency of these various nutrients can cause a breakdown in health. Naturopaths and herbalists consider blackstrap molasses a vital nutritive food for treating a wide range of disorders, including circulatory problems and heart trouble.

Molasses may be taken before, during, or after meals. Cyril Scott of England suggests the dosage of one teaspoonful dissolved in half a cup of hot water, then cold water added to make two-thirds of a cupful, and the mixture sipped slowly. For children, half the dosage. Anyone with a sensitive stomach who finds one teaspoonful too much at one time may take a smaller dose more often during the day.

High Blood Pressure

Mrs. G. S. of South Africa writes:

"I would like to tell you of the experience we had with my mother. She had suffered with high blood pressure for over twenty years. Two years ago she was in the hospital after a terrible nosebleed which couldn't be stopped. This was probably a godsend at the time.

"After discharge from the hospital she was asked to attend outpatients' clinic once a month to have her blood pressure checked, and was given treatment, three pills a day. In spite of this, her pressure continued extremely high—once touching 240.

"One day my young son walked in with a very large jar of crude blackstrap molasses which he had obtained from a cane company. He had read of its effectiveness in high blood pressure. My mother has taken a small teaspoon of this in a tea-cup of hot water before breakfast and supper every day. It wasn't nice at first, but she has grown accustomed to the taste.

"Since she started this ten months ago, her blood pressure has been completely normal each time it has been tested. Doctor's pills have been gradually reduced to two a day, then one a day, and now will go to one in three days.

"I do hope some of your readers will be helped."

Varicose Veins

The condition of varicose veins is a common complaint. Medical herbalists warn that in this condition small clots of blood may form if the blood flow stops sufficiently. This can give rise to phlebitis (inflammation of a vein). In such cases the leg should never be massaged as there may be a loosely attached blood clot which could travel up to the heart or lungs, and cause a dangerous situation to arise.

Blackstrap molasses has proved successful in treating varicose veins, according to many people who have used it. For example, one woman wrote that she suffered from this condition for more than 50 years. The veins had become so enlarged that she could not straighten her legs in bed. She had consulted several doctors who stated that in their entire practice they had never seen such a severe condition of varicose veins. They advised her to have them surgically removed, but she refused. At the suggestion of an acquaintance, she tried blackstrap molasses, not expecting it would do any good. She reported that after taking it for several weeks, she awoke one morning to find to her astonishment that the condition of the diseased veins had completely vanished.

Heart Trouble

The ingredients in blackstrap molasses are very beneficial for the health of the heart. Tachycardia, arteriosclerosis, weak heart, cardiac thrombosis (blood clot), and a number of other heart problems have reportedly responded to treatment with blackstrap molasses.

Strokes

According to medical herbalists, many strokes have yielded to the use of blackstrap molasses. It has been shown that where paralysis results from a stroke, there was a lack of calcium, magnesium, and potassium in the body. All these minerals are contained in blackstrap molasses.

NOTE: Diabetics should not use molasses.

HONEY

Herbalists recommend two teaspoons of honey at each mealtime for controlling cramp in the legs or feet. Generally the cramp disappears within a week, but the honey should be continued daily to prevent a return of the difficulty.

Honey for the Heart

Dr. G. N. W. Thomas of Edinburgh, Scotland writes:

"In heart weakness I have found honey to have a marked effect in reviving the heart action and keeping patients alive. I had further evidence of this in a recent case of pneumonia. The patient consumed two pounds of honey during the illness; there was an early crisis with no subsequent rise of temperature and an exceptionally good pulse. I suggest that honey should be given for general physical repair, and above all for heart failure."

Sir Arbuthnot Lane regards honey as a valuable heart and muscle stimulant, and an excellent source of energy. In his opinion there is no better food for muscular fatigue and exhaustion.

Dr. Arnold Lorand refers to the value of honey as follows:

"As the best food for the heart, I recommend honey. Honey is easily digested and assimilated; it is the best sweet food, as it does not cause flatulence and can prevent it, to a certain extent promoting the activity of the bowels. It can easily be added to the five meals a day I recommend in cases of arteriosclerosis and for weak heart."

In some countries, herbalists consider honey to be an effective remedy for dispersing fluid from around the heart. Two teaspoons of honey are taken three times a day with meals.

COMFREY

Botanical Name: *Symphytum officinalis*
Common Name: Knitbone, Common Comfrey

Among its many uses, comfrey is highly valued by herbalists as a remedy for varicose ulcers. For this condition, poultices or compresses are prepared from the boiled cut roots of the herb, and applied to the affected area. Or comfrey ointment may be used instead.

Case Histories

Many case histories attest to the healing qualities of comfrey for treating varicose ulcers. Here is a sampling:

• "Some years ago, I suffered from a nasty varicose ulcer, which refused to heal in spite of a number of different medications that were tried. My physician told me to keep off my legs as much as possible, which helped relieve the pain, but still the ulcer did not heal. My cousin corresponds with a dear friend in England, and she mentioned my problem to her. The lady wrote back and suggested trying comfrey poultices. The remedy worked miracles. Within two months the ulcer had completely healed."—Mrs. L. I.

• "I had a very painful varicose ulcer for more than five years. One day I read where comfrey was used with wonderful success in treating bed sores. It seemed to me that if it could heal such stubborn conditions, it might work for my leg ulcer. So in desperation I tried it. I boiled the roots, and when the tea had cooled I soaked a piece of gauze in it and lightly bound the compress directly on the ulcer. This was done several times daily, making sure the compress was always kept moist and not allowed to dry out. I was truly amazed to see the improvement as the days went by, and in a few short weeks the ulcer was gone!"–J.R.

• Ms. K. P. wrote that her friend told her their family doctor wanted to amputate her mother's leg as gangrene had set in from a varicose ulcer she had had for seven years. Medical treatment in and out of the hospital had failed to heal the ulcer during that time. Ms. K. P. says she told her friend all about the healing properties of comfrey and suggested she try comfrey poultices on her mother's leg. She also suggested that her mother be given cups of comfrey tea to drink, several times a day. These suggestions were followed with the cooperation of the district nurse who had attended to the prescribed dressings over the past years, and also that of her medically trained son. Ms. K. P. says:

"Within a week, signs that the skin surrounding the open sore was beginning to heal were observed, and within three months the whole sore had healed completely. This so impressed the nurse that she then decided to try the treatment on another of her patients who had had varicose ulcers for 17 years. Naturally, these sores have taken longer, but after eight months they are almost healed."

Ms. K. P. explains that the poultices cause considerable itching, which is believed due to the rapid healing process. It was found that the use of comfrey ointment does not cause itching, but it is slower in its healing action.

HOW PROPER DIET CAN HELP PROTECT AGAINST HEART ATTACKS

International medical research has shown that people who consume magnesium-rich foods have lower incidences of heart disease. Studies in England, Finland, and Canada (where water and soil are both low in magnesium content) revealed that victims who died of sudden heart attacks had levels of magnesium that averaged 12 to 17 percent lower than normal. In one of these studies, Dr. T.W. Anderson of the University of British Columbia discovered that the amount of magnesium in the heart muscle of people who died of sudden heart attacks was about 30 percent below normal.

According to Dr. Barton Altura, a heart expert, magnesium protects you from blood vessels overcontracting and causing a heart attack. He believes that 50 to 75 percent of all fatal sudden heart attacks could be prevented in men between the ages of 20 and 50, by taking proper amounts of magnesium. He adds that even patients being treated for heart attacks could benefit from magnesium.

Dr. Mildred Seeling, M.D., also points out that research has shown that you can protect yourself from sudden heart attacks with adequate amounts of magnesium.

Other researchers have confirmed these findings. For example, as a result of studies conducted by Dr. Carl Johnson on men who died of sudden heart attacks, he found there was a direct connection between magnesium deficiencies and the risk of dying of a heart attack. He said that people can reduce their chance of having a heart attack by keeping their levels of magnesium up in their daily diet. This can be done by eating natural foods such as raw green vegetables, whole grains, cereals, nuts, beans, fish, and seafood. Or a person can take magnesium supplements which are available from most health food stores, herb firms, and pharmacies, and are non-toxic according to experts. However, it is pointed out that if you have any severe medical problem such as kidney disease, your doctor should be consulted first.

Although the U.S. National Academy of Science has been recommending 350 milligrans of magnesium daily, Dr. Altura believes that people need more—about 400 to 500 milligrams per day.

SUMMARY

1. Palpitation or tachycardia is one of the most common of the many different types of heart trouble.
2. In the herbal system of medicine, hawthorn berry is regarded as a top-ranking botanical for numerous heart conditions.
3. Extensive research by a number of medical teams has shown that a cholesterol-lowering diet is a prime factor in preventing arteriosclerosis.
4. Scientific findings from all parts of the world have revealed that garlic is a near specific remedy for high blood pressure.
5. British doctors have demonstrated that the humble onion can help prevent or dissolve deadly internal blood clots.
6. International medical research has discovered that people who consume magnesium-rich foods have lower incidences of heart disease.
7. Crude blackstrap molasses is very rich in minerals and also contains most of the B vitamins. Natural practitioners consider it to be a vital nutritive food for treating many disorders,

including heart trouble and circulatory problems. However, it should not be used by diabetics.

8. There are many other natural aids that have proven effective for coping with various circulatory and heart ailments.

CHAPTER 9

Herbs for Treating Female Disorders

There are a number of different ailments that can affect women, as for example, menstrual difficulties, premenstrual tension, vaginal inflammation and discharge, ovarian cysts, urethral irritation, vomiting during pregnancy, miscarriage, and so on. Premenstrual tension may cause symptoms such as crying jags, depression, headaches, tender breasts, water retention, insomnia, constipation, and bloating. Statistics have shown that at this time women drink more alcohol, commit more crimes, have higher suicide attempts, and are more accident prone.

In older women, the stress of the menopause may bring about a swarm of insidious symptoms, such as hot flashes, irritability, a kind of rheumatism known as "menopausal arthritis," or that dismal depression popularly called "menopausal melancholia." It is difficult for many women going through the menopause to be sparkling and cheerful.

HERB REMEDIES FOR COPING WITH FEMALE DISORDERS

Herbs are used in different parts of the world to relieve or eliminate various female problems and to improve female health the natural way.

LADY'S MANTLE

Botanical Name: *Alchemilla vulgaris*
Common Names: Lion's Foot, Bear's Foot

This is a perennial plant which bears numerous small, yellow-green flowers. In the Middle Ages it was associated with the Virgin Mary, because the leaves were said to resemble the scalloped edges of a mantle. In Latin it was called *Leontopodium* (lion's foot) due to its spreading root-leaves, and in modern French this has become *Pied-de-lion*. Lady's mantle is known in German as *Frauenmantle*.

The generic name, Alchemilla, is derived from the Arabic word *Alkemelch* (alchemy), and according to some of the early writers was given to the plant because of its wondrous powers.

Lady's mantle contains astringent and styptic properties, and is used in modern herbal medicine as a remedy for profuse menstruation. It is prepared as a tea, one ounce to one pint of boiling water. The tea is steeped for ten minutes, then strained. It is taken in teacupful doses as required. In Sweden, a tincture of the leaves is used, one-half to one teaspoonful in a small glass of water three times a day.

A strong decoction of lady's mantle root used as a douche is reputed to be a good remedy for the condition of leucorrhea.

Menopausal Melancholia

Lady's mantle is combined with other herbs as a remedy for menopausal melancholia. One ounce each of lady's mantle, red raspberry leaves, and lime flowers are thoroughly mixed together. Two teaspoonfuls of the mixture are placed in a teapot and one pint of boiling water is added. The tea is allowed to steep for ten minutes, then strained. One teacupful is taken as needed.

PEACH TREE

Botanical Name: *Prunus persica*
Common Name: Peach Tree

The peach tree is native to China, a fact which is shown by the Chinese character representing it—one of the few unchanged ancient Chinese characters. It was mentioned in the books of

Confucius in the fifth century, and representations of it appeared in sculpture and on porcelain.

The peach has been cultivated in most parts of Asia, and is said to have been introduced into Europe from Persia, as part of its botanical name, *Persica*, implies. The Romans brought it from Persia during the reign of the Emperor Claudius, but it was not introduced into England until the sixteenth century.

Many different parts of the peach tree are highly valued in Chinese herbal medicine for coping with various ailments. It is especially considered to be a very good remedy for preventing or relieving the nausea and vomiting of morning sickness (vomiting during pregnancy). Two to four tablespoonfuls of the tea are taken first thing in the morning, and the same dosage continued if necessary every one or two hours, or oftener. It reputedly acts very promptly to bring relief in most cases.

The tea may be prepared the night before. One pint of boiling water is poured over one and a half ounces of dried peach leaves. The container is covered with a lid, and the tea allowed to stand until cold. It is then strained and stored overnight in the refrigerator. In the morning the tea is reheated and taken warm according to the dosages previously cited.

Variations of the Peach Remedy

Peach remedies for relieving morning sickness are also very popular in many parts of Europe. Some prefer the use of a decoction prepared with one-half ounce of the bark to one pint of boiling water. This is simmered slowly for ten minutes, then strained. It is taken in doses of a tablespoonful to a wineglassful as required. Others prefer an infusion: one ounce of the leaves is placed in a container with one pint of water. As soon as the water boils, the container is immediately removed from the burner and the tea allowed to stand until cold. It is then strained, reheated, and taken warm in doses of a tablespoon to a wineglassful as needed.

Dr. Eric Powell of England presents the following:

Peach medicine is undoubtedly one of the best remedies for the vomiting of pregnancy. This is probably due to its very soothing effect on the gastric surfaces. We have known many cases of distressed pregnant females finding immediate benefit from this simple remedy. It must be pointed out that there are some who do not respond to the infusion of the dried plant; these usually react right away to the fresh plant tincture of the bark, for which the dose is about five drops in a little tepid water. As a rule, the infusion will prove to be satisfactory.

RED RASPBERRY

Botanical Name: *Rubus strigosus*
Common Name: Red Raspberry

This is a shrubby plant which grows in many parts of the world, including the uplands of the central and western provinces of China. Its Chinese name, Fu-p'en-tzu, means "a turned-over bowl" in reference to the fruit.

In herbal medicine, raspberry leaf tea is used as a female tonic and restorative. It is employed to help prevent miscarriage, to relieve the severe labor pains of childbirth, and to treat urethral irritation and menstrual difficulties.

English herbalists have long prescribed raspberry leaf tea for pregnant women. They have found that in most cases it helps prevent miscarriage and ensures an easy labor. For this use the expectant mother takes a pint of the raspberry leaf tea daily. This is made by placing one ounce of dried raspberry leaves in a porcelain container and pouring on them a pint of boiling water. The tea is covered and allowed to stand until cold, then strained. A small cupful of the reheated tea is taken half an hour before each meal. It may be sweetened with a little honey.

In reference to the use of raspberry leaf tea, Dr. Fox stated that it was an excellent remedy for the relief of painful and profuse menstruation, and to regulate the labor pains of women in childbirth.

Case Histories

• J. H. Oliver, a medical herbalist of England, reported: "A lady doctor who had been practicing for many years in a maternity home, and had helped thousands of babies into the world, told us she had always insisted that the prospective mothers take raspberry leaf tea, and she scorned the idea of ever losing a case. Since we started this campaign we have received scores of letters from grateful parents. One lady told us she was reading the paper only a few minutes before her baby was born."

• A Canadian herbalist presents the following information on red raspberry leaf tea: "Red raspberry leaves: a good source of vitamins A, B, C, G and E. They are rich in calcium, phosphorus, iron, and an unknown factor that prevents miscarriage.

I know of several cases where this was proved beyond a doubt. A woman had four miscarriages, and despaired of ever bearing a child. Several doctors told her that she could never become a mother. On advice given by close members of my family, she took to drinking raspberry leaf tea every morning during pregnancy. She gave birth to a lovely girl, and in eighteen months she had another. The labor in both cases was practically painless."

• Here is another interesting account which appeared in an English health publication: "A number of people find it difficult to relax when nervous or in pain, women particularly, especially during childbirth. The birth of my own first child was prolonged and frightening, mainly due to my fear and inability to relax the necessary muscles.

"Three years later, when I was pregnant again, I dreaded the coming ordeal. I had not, as yet, discovered the benefits of herbs. One day I was admiring a sow and litter with a neighboring farmer and remarked on the dreadfulness of producing such a large family. He laughed and told me that he always gave his sows an herbal remedy of raspberry leaf tea to help them when farrowing, and also thought that many ladies could benefit from the same herb.

"I was willing to try anything to allay my fears, and purchased a packet of raspberry leaf tea from a local herbalist. At first I did not care for its unusual flavor but in time I grew accustomed to it, and schooled myself to take it regularly. The months passed and the day came when I knew my baby would soon arrive. I was filled with an apprehension, which I soon found was quite unnecessary. My fears vanished when I found myself responding quite involuntarily to the muscular contractions with very little discomfort, and was amazed when the baby came into the world with such ease. My crowning achievement was a lovely little daughter whose quick arrival forestalled a surprised doctor who remembered my last drawn-out ordeal.

"The practical experience with herbal treatment has strengthened my belief in the potential cures that are obtained from herbs. I have since learned that Dr. Grantley Dick Read advocated the use of raspberry leaf tea as an aid to easier childbirth in some of his studies of natural childbirth.

"So the farmer's recommendation proved successful; only someone who has suffered pain because of unrelaxed muscles can know the advantage of discovering a reliable source of help, and a simple one, too.

"I am fully convinced that I found such a remedy in

raspberry leaf tea, and by taking it regularly throughout the latter months of pregnancy ensured myself of an easier birth."

Combined Formulas

Red raspberry is often combined with other herbs for treating various female disorders.

For Ovarian Cysts: One ounce each of raspberry leaves, black currant leaves, witch hazel leaves and powdered myrrh are boiled in one quart of water in a covered container for five minutes, then simmered slowly for one-half hour. It is then strained, and a quarter of a pint of this mixture is added to a pint of cold water and used as a douche nightly. In addition, a tea is prepared with one ounce each of comfrey root, yellow dock root, yarrow root and dandelion root, with two ounces of licorice root. The herbs are thoroughly mixed and divided into three equal parts. To one part, a pint of boiling water is added, and simmered slowly for ten minutes. It is then cooled, strained, and a tablespoonful taken three or four times daily.

To Relieve the Condition of Leucorrhea: One ounce each of the fluid extract or tincture of raspberry leaves, gentian root, golden seal, and comfrey are mixed together in one bottle. One teaspoonful of the combined fluid extract or tincture is taken in a little water three times daily.

In addition to taking the above formula, the cleansing process of an herbal douche is used. A mixture of one ounce each of raspberry leaves, white oak bark, witch hazel leaves, black current leaves and cranesbill herb is boiled slowly in two quarts of water for 20 minutes, then strained through a cloth. The straining process should be continued until the liquid is perfectly clear, and when the solution has cooled to a tepid warm it is used as a douche. A fresh batch should be prepared and used every other night until the condition has cleared up. Some cases respond favorably after one or two douches; others require longer treatments of a week or ten days and even longer. However, once the leucorrhea has stopped, the douches should not be continued.

AMARANTH

Botanical Name: *Amaranthus hypochondriacus*
Common Names: Prince's Feather, Velvet Flower, Red Cock's Comb

This is an annual herb with an upright stem from three to four feet high. It has bright reddish-purple, clustering flowers of a plume-like form, and is grown as an ornamental plant in gardens.

In folklore, this flower is regarded as the symbol of immortality. The name is taken from the Greek *amarantos*, meaning "incorruptible." It was the practice among the Greeks to spread the flowers of amaranth over the graves of the dead to demonstrate their belief in the immortality of the soul.

Medicinal Use of Amaranth

Amaranth contains a generous amount of vitamins and minerals, and in France its leaves are cooked and eaten in place of spinach.

For centuries the plant has been employed as a remedy for profuse menstruation. The early herbalists also employed it in the treatment of diarrhea and dysentery. Dr. O. Phelps Brown wrote an account of the herb in which he stated that the plant is an astringent, and said: "The decoction drunk freely is highly useful in severe menorrhagia [profuse menstruation], in diarrhea, dysentery, etc."

Drs. Wood and Ruddock also classified the herb as an astringent: "This herb is most noted as an effectual cure for profuse menstruation for which purpose a tea is to be drunk freely, four or five times a day. It is an astringent, and as such it is also used in bowel complaints."

The tea is prepared by placing two ounces of the herb in a container and adding one quart of boiling water. The brew is covered, allowed to stand until cold, then strained. The tea is reheated to take the chill off, and one large cup of the lukewarm tea is taken four or five times a day. (In more severe cases, the tea is taken more often.)

If a fluid extract of the herb is used, the dose is one-half to one teaspoonful in a little water three or four times a day.

Reported Use

• "I suffered from excessive bleeding during my periods. My doctor's exam showed nothing functionally wrong. However, not only was I frightened by the loss of so much blood, but unless I was very careful it could cause me terrible embarrassment when in public. One time while attending a women's garden club meeting I suddenly felt my period starting. As I got up to go to the dressing room I learned that the whole seat of my dress was stained with blood. The other women were very sympathetic, but I was humiliated beyond words.

"Later at another of these meetings one of the members told me of a remedy that her grandmother had used for excessive menstruation when she was young. She said it was an herb tea called amaranth, and assured me that it was perfectly harmless. I drank the tea as instructed, a couple of days before and during my next period. The results were wonderful, there was no flooding! I continue to drink the tea every month, and wouldn't think of being without it."—Mrs. L. J.

WHITE ASH

Botanical Name: *Fraxinus americana*
Common Name: White Ash

The white ash tree is chiefly found in the Northern United States and Canada. It is a large forest tree, growing to great height. Due to the excellent quality of its wood it was used in the past to make bows and arrows, agricultural tools, wagons, railway carriages, and so on.

Medicinal Use

Around the turn of the century, Dr. Compton Burnett, M.D., the famous English homeopathic physician-author, found that a tincture prepared from white ash tree bark acted specifically on the uterus. He found it particularly helpful in dissolving fibrous uterine growths and curing prolapse of the uterus.

In several of his books, Dr. Burnett gives many case histories of patients treated for tumors and prolapse. For example, one woman, age 38, already the mother of six children, came to him with the diagnosis of a greatly enlarged uterus which had to be propped up with a pessary. Although she had been told she must have surgery to correct this condition, Dr. Burnett persuaded her to give his medical treatment a trial. She was told to take five drops of tincture of *Fraxinus* (white ash) three times daily in water. A week later the woman felt so much better she decided not to have the operation. Seven weeks later, still taking the tincture, the woman, who had not been able to walk without discomfort and back pain, went to Scotland and took long walks on the moors without any adverse effects.

Following Dr. Burnett's lead, other physicians in England used *Fraxinus* in their practice, reportedly with great success. One such doctor tells of a 75-year-old patient who had prolapse of the uterus and vagina with bearing-down pains. She was given the tincture, five drops three times daily, and in spite of her advanced age the ligaments tightened and drew up the prolapsed organ.

DONG QUAI

Botanical Name: *Angelica polymorphoa*
Common Name: Dong Quai

In different parts of China, according to the variations of dialect, this Oriental plant is called either Dong Quai or Tang Kwei. Botanically, the herb is known as *Angelica polymorpha*, but is often mistaken by Westerners as either common angelica (*Angelica archangelica*) or Lovage (*Ligusticum*).

Dong Quai root is famed in Chinese medicine for its affinity for the female constitution. It is highly valued as a remedy for nourishing female glands, regulating monthly periods, relieving menstrual cramps, and correcting menopausal symptoms.

How Dong Quai Is Used

Powdered Dong Quai is available in capsules which may be swallowed with a glass of hot water, or broken open and the contents added to hot soups or broths. Since its taste somewhat resembles that of celery, it adds to, rather than detracts from, the flavor of various food dishes.

For best results, little or no fruit or fruit juices should be taken while using Dong Quai. Vegetables should be included in the diet, and cooked with a slice of ginger root.

Compounded Dong Quai

In addition to the regular Dong Quai capsules which are prepared from the upper parts of a *single* root, there is a super type of powdered Chinese Dong Quai also available in capsule form which is a processed compound prepared from the upper parts of *several* roots. If the regular Dong Quai capsules are used, women generally take two capsules three times a day; if the stronger Chinese Super Compounded type is used, only two capsules are taken daily, one in the morning and one in the

evening. In very severe cases, two capsules of the Super Compounded type may be taken twice or three times daily until the
condition improves, at which time the dosage is reduced to one
capsule twice a day.

The processed Super Dong Quai Compound also comes in
the form of hard, compressed nuggets (shaped somewhat like
marshmallows) which are wrapped in cellophane pouches and
packed in a box. A tea is made by placing one of the nuggets in
a cup and adding boiling water. The nugget quickly dissolves as
the tea is stirred. Two or three cups of the tea are taken daily.

Reported Uses

• A young mother writes: "Both my teenage daughter and I
used to suffer every month from menstrual troubles, until we
found out about Chinese Dong Quai. When the time for my
daughter's period rolled around she would get cramps and turn
very pale, and it took several days for the menstruation to begin.
Now she swallows two Super Dong Quai capsules with a cup of
hot water as soon as her cramps begin, with the result that the
flow starts and her pains subside. As for myself, I had a different
set of symptoms: several days before my period was due my
stomach became bloated, I suffered from headaches, and then
when the period did start I got terrible grinding cramps which
lasted the entire first day. I always had to go to bed with a hot
water bottle on my abdomen. However when I began taking
Super Dong Quai I was able to avoid all these unpleasant
symptoms. I require more of the Dong Quai than my daughter—at
least three capsules per day until my period is well established.
We both find it quite a relief, for as any woman knows, it's no
fun to go through a lot of misery every 28 days."

• Mrs. B. W., age 55, writes: "When I started into the menopause I seemed to have every classic symptom of it that I'd ever
heard about. I was irritable and depressed, very sensitive to my
surroundings, feeling every little draught or change of temperature, and noise bothered me considerably. Physically I was
deteriorating too, with miserable hot flashes, and twinges of
rheumatism in my hands and feet. My complexion was drawn
and pale, and there were dark circles under my eyes. However,
there was nothing wrong with my perseverance, as I kept
doggedly trying to find something to help me. I didn't want to
take injections of estrogen as I felt that was an invitation to
serious side effects. Finally a Chinese lady I worked with

suggested I try Dong Quai as she said it was a favorite with Oriental women going through the menopause. I began taking two, and sometimes three, capsules of the Super Compounded type of Dong Quai daily, and within two weeks was feeling sweeter tempered and more relaxed. As the months passed, the unpleasant physical and emotional symptoms disappeared completely and I began feeling healthier than I had in many years. Family and friends noticed how much better I looked. I suffered no further trouble whatever from the menopause so long as I kept taking those wonderful Dong Quai capsules. Please pass the good word along to other women."

• "A teen-age girl missed her monthly period for six months. She had been taken to a medical doctor, but her condition did not improve. Her parents were very worried and finally took the girl to a Chinese herbalist who prescribed a bottle of Compounded Dong Quai capsules. A few days later the parents went back to the herbalist and happily reported that their daughter's period had started. They saw him again a year later and informed him that the girl had never had any further trouble with her periods." —Mrs. L.S.

• "Dissolving a nugget of Super Dong Quai in a cup of hot water and drinking the tea is the best remedy in the world for menstrual cramps. I know of three other women besides myself who have found blessed relief from monthly cramps with this remarkable remedy." —Miss B.B.

• "Let me tell you how Dong Quai has taken care of my problem when my gynecologist couldn't. For several months I had a little bleeding between my monthly periods. I had noticed my periods were arriving sooner, lasted longer, and I was bleeding more. I had consulted my gynecologist several times and after thorough check-ups I was told there was nothing medically wrong with me to cause this abnormality, but that if it occurred again, I could easily be put on hormones, have a scraping or a hysterectomy (but I was also told I was too young to have any of these). But then I bled for 15 days and was afraid to call my doctor again and to face the same answer or an operation. So I took Super Compounded Dong Quai capsules for a month and everything was fine! I took the capsules for one more month, and now five months have passed and I have no menstrual problems whatsoever. I am back to normal, thanks to Dong Quai."
—Mrs Y. L.

SUMMARY

1. There are various ailments that can affect the human female.
2. In older women, the stress of the menopause can bring about a swarm of insidious symptoms such as irritability, hot flashes, dismal depression, and menopausal rheumatism.
3. Herb remedies are used in many parts of the world for coping with female disorders, and for building female health the natural way.
4. Chinese Dong Quai is available in powdered form prepared from the upper parts of a single root, and as a stronger compound prepared from the upper parts of several roots.
5. For best results, little or no fruit or fruit juice should be taken while using Dong Quai as these would neutralize the beneficial effects of the herbal compound. Vegetables should be included in the diet, cooked with a slice of ginger root.
6. When drinking herb teas for leuchorrhea, herbal douches are also used as an accessory treatment.

CHAPTER 10

Nature's Health Secrets for Coping with Men's Ailments

Following is a list of plant remedies used in Europe and other lands for treating various ailments that affect the human male.

PUMPKIN

Botanical Name: *Cucurbita maxima*
Common Name: Pumpkin

Pumpkin seeds have been used for their beneficial effects on the prostate gland. This is an old time folk-remedy which has been handed down from one generation to another. It should be of considerable interest to every man, since medical science informs us that some difficulty with the prostate gland affects almost every American male over the age of fifty. Physicians explain that during this period of life, the prostate gland may swell and cause extreme difficulty of urination. Eventually it may be impossible to urinate due to pressure of the gland upon the bladder, and the use of a catheter for withdrawal of the urine will be required. The accumulation of urine in the bladder may consequently cause infection.

Dr. W. Devrient of Germany believes that prevention is the best course to follow with regard to prostate trouble. He says that in certain countries where pumpkin seeds are consumed in abundance throughout life, there is practically no incidence of prostate disorders. Dr. Devrient writes:

"Only the plain people knew of the open secret of pumpkin seeds—a secret which was handed down from father to son for countless generations without any ado. No matter whether it was the Hungarian gypsy, the mountain-dwelling Bulgarian, the Anatolian Turk, the Ukranian, the Transylvanian German—they all knew that pumpkin seeds preserve the prostate gland and thereby also male potency. In these countries, people eat pumpkin seeds the way they eat sunflower seeds in Russia—as an inexhaustible source of vigor offered by Nature.

"Investigations by G. Klein at the Vienna University revealed the noteworthy fact that in Transylvania prostatic hypertrophy is almost unknown. Painstaking researches result in the disclosure that the people there have a special liking for pumpkin seeds. A physician from the Szekler group in the Transylvanian mountains confirmed this connection as an ancient healing method among the people. Dr. Bela Pater of Klausenburg later published these associations and his own experiences in the *Journal of Healing and Seasoning Plants*.

"My assertion of the androgen-hormonal [the male hormone] influence of pumpkin seeds is based on the positive judgment of old-time doctors, but also no less on my own personal observation throughout the years. This plant has scientifically determined effects on intermediary metabolism and diuresis [urination], but these latter are of secondary importance in relation to its regenerative, invigorative, and vitalizing influences. There is involved herein a native plant hormone which affects our own hormone production in part by substitution, in part by direct proliferation.

"Anyone who has studied this influence among peasant peoples has been again and again astonished over the effect of this plant in putting off the advent of old age. My own personal observations in the course of the last eight years, however, have been decisive for me. At my own age of 70 years I am well able to be satisfied with the condition of my own prostate, on the basis of daily ingestion of pumpkin seeds and with that of my health in general. This beneficial result can also be found among city patients who are prudent enough to eat pumpkin seeds every day and throughout life. But one must continue proving this to the city dweller. The peasants of the Balkans and of Eastern Europe knew of the healing effects of these seeds already from their forefathers."

Valuable Nutrients in Pumpkin Seeds

Drs. Julian Grant and Henry Feinblatt discovered an important new medication consisting of three amino acids, which brought about prompt and dramatic relief for patients suffering from enlarged prostate associated with urinary difficulties. Pumpkin seeds contain the very same amino acids.

Chemical analyses of the healthy prostate gland show very high concentration of zinc, whereas the amount of this mineral in the sick prostate is low. This seems to indicate that zinc is extremely important to the health of the prostate.

Pumpkin seeds are one of the richest natural sources of zinc.

Magnesium is another important mineral found abundantly in pumpkin seeds. Several medical doctors in France have achieved remarkable results in the prevention and cure of prostate disorders by administering magnesium compounds. One French physician, Dr. Chevassu, treated twelve prostatic patients with the compound, and reported that ten of the twelve patients were completely cured and their general physical health also greatly improved.

Another French physician made inquiries of some of his male colleagues who took a magnesium compound after they had read a report of its effectiveness in treating prostate trouble. He learned that four out of five of them had suffered difficulty in urinating, but after using the magnesium tablets, their urinating problems had greatly lessened or disappeared completely.

SAW PALMETTO

Botanical Name: *Sabal serrulata*
Common Name: Sabal

This plant or shrub grows best along the southeastern coast of the United States, and can be found extending inland eight or ten miles. The nearer to the sea, the more luxuriant is its growth. Saw palmetto produces dark purple berries about the size of an olive.

Remedial Uses

This plant is classed as diuretic, stimulant, and tonic. Liquid preparations of the berries are used for numerous complaints, but are especially valued for their reputed ability to provide nutrition to the testicles in functional atrophy of those organs. Saw palmetto also has a longstanding reputation as a remedy for prostate trouble. For any of these conditions, preparations of the berries are generally combined with one or more other appropriate botanicals.

Dr. Eric Powell writes: "Quite recently I had an elderly gentleman who had been ordered to have an operation for enlarged prostate. He passed urine with great difficulty. Doses of five drops of the combined tinctures of Echinacea and Sabal [saw palmetto berries] normalized the gland in three months. I was particularly pleased with the result in this case owing to his age, for he was over seventy!"

In reference to echinacea in the above formula, Dr. Powell says it is one of the best herbal alteratives, and has a marked affinity for the prostate gland in conditions of weakness or enlargement of that organ.

Dr. Yemm suggests a combination of one ounce each of the fluid extracts of saw palmetto berries, damiana, and kola nut, for "nervous and sexual debility." He recommends one teaspoon of the mixture in a small glass of water, three times daily before meals, and advises that the diet be light and easily digestible.

POLLEN

A fine powder, usually yellow in color, forms inside the blossoms of herbs and flowers and is commonly known as pollen.

In Norse mythology it was believed that pagan gods ate a secret food called ambrosia, which accounted for their immortality. Ambrosia was a combination of bee bread and honey, which is another name for pollen stored in honeycomb cells. According to ancient texts of Egypt, China, Babylon, and Persia it was agreed that this valuable plant substance was the magic key to the secret of health, strength, and longevity.

Today in many regions of the world, the eating of pollen is still practiced. Island natives cherish pollen as a youth sustainer and as an effective remedy for many ills. It is said that the natives of the Burma jungles remain virile, energetic, and healthy right up into advanced years. An important part of their daily diet is pollen-honey cakes, and they also keep a supply of powdered pollen on hand for medicinal purposes.

Nicolai Tsitsin, a Russian biologist, investigated ways of prolonging human life. He was impressed to discover that a number of people in Russia who claimed to be over 100 years of age had consumed pollen as the principal food of their diet.

In many lands pollen is used as a remedy for impotence and prostate trouble.

Valuable Constituents in Pollen

Two European universities termed pollen one of the richest food substances, saying that it is "without equal in Nature."

An analysis by scientific researchers in Switzerland reveals that pollen contains free amino acids, various forms of sugar, mucilage, fats, minerals, protein, trace elements, hormone components, large quantities of the vitamin B. complex, and also vitamins A, D, E, and C.

The Health Benefits of Pollen

Dr. Ask-Upmark of Sweden reported on a case of prostate infection that he had been unable to completely cure in five years of orthodox treatment. One day the patient decided on his own initiative to take pollen tablets as he felt he needed something to strengthen his general condition. He took six tablets daily, and Dr. Ask-Upmark says the improvement in his prostate condition was like a miracle. The patient had only one recurrence of the trouble, and that was due to the fact that he neglected to take the pollen tablets for two weeks. Once he began taking the tablets every day again, he had no further prostate trouble.

Later, Dr. Ask-Upmark treated 12 cases of prostatitis (inflammation of the prostate gland) with a dosage of five to six pollen tablets daily, taken first thing in the morning. Ten of the 12 patients showed remarkable improvement. Of the two cases that did not, one was due to another medical complication. The other engaged in the sport of salmon fishing and as a result would go wading up to his knees in the icy cold Norwegian rivers. Dr. Ask-Upmark felt that this wading aggravated the prostate condition, and since the patient would not give up the habit, pollen treatment was discontinued.

Professor Izet Osmanagic, head of the Gynecological Department at the University of Sarajevo, reported the result of his trials with a strong blend of pollen and royal jelly on 40 men, aged 20 to 52. He found that 75 percent of the men suffered from poor sperm production and partial impotence. All the patients had had sterile marriages for two or more years.

The patients took two capsules of the pollen blend daily, and when the course of two or three months of treatment ended, each had taken a total of either 80 or 120 capsules.

After one month, more than half of the patients had improved in their sexual and general condition. One fourth found that their cohabitation ability had improved, and the majority showed improvement of sperm production. Two of the men were happy to announce that their wives were pregnant.

Professor Heise of the Urological Clinic of Magdeburg treated nine prostate patients with pollen extract, one tablet three times a day. All had similar symptoms, e.g., difficulty in urinating, pain, lowered libido, painful orgasms, bacterially positive emissions, difficulty during coitus, and some showed manifestations of impotence. Dr. Heise reported that when the course of treatment had ended, all the patients had responded with definite improvement. He concluded that it would be commendable if treatment with pollen preparation were to be incorporated into recommended therapeutic practice.

Dr. L. J. Denis, a urologist in Antwerp, Belgium, selected ten patients who suffered prostatitis but in whom no evidence of infection was detected. They all experienced discomfort when urinating. Four had pain in one of the testicles, groin, or perineum, and three complained of loss of sexual desire. The ten patients were treated with four pollen extract tablets daily. At the end of the treatment, the patients said they had improved and no longer complained of their symptoms.

Alken, Jonsson, and Rohl, a distinguished German-Swedish urological team, treated 172 cases of prostatitis with a pollen preparation. They found that relief was produced in 44% of the cases, which they felt was very satisfactory.

SEA HOLLY

Botanical Name: : *Eryngium maritimum*
Common Name: Eryngo

This plant grows abundantly on the sandy coasts of Europe. The leaves have a sea-green hue and are veined with white; the thistle-like flowers are fringed with blue. It is regarded as a beautiful ornamental plant and is cultivated in gardens. In olden times sea holly had the legendary reputation of causing faithfulness in husbands, if worn by their wives.

Remedial Uses

Among its many uses, sea holly is regarded as a good remedy for certain conditions affecting the male organs. A medical herbalist of England mentions the case of a young boy who suffered from hydrocele (a collection of fluid in a sac surrounding the testicle). A physician had informed the boy's mother that an operation was necessary, but she decided to see if an herbal practitioner could help, before submitting her son to surgery. The herbalist prescribed the following mixture:

>Fluid extract of Eryngo (Sea Holly), one ounce.
>Fluid extract of Symphytum (Comfrey), 4 dr.
>Five-drop dose—three times a day.

He reports that later the boy was examined by the physician, and the mother was informed there was nothing further to worry about as the hydrocele condition had disappeared. The condition never returned.

DAMIANA

Botanical Name: : *Turnera aphrodisiaca*
Common Name: Mexican Damiana

This is a small shrub bearing aromatic yellowish flowers. It is indigenous to Mexico, South America, Lower California, Texas, and the West Indies.

Remedial Uses

In the Mexican pharmacopeia, damiana is classed as aphrodisiac, diuretic, and tonic. In that country it has been scientifically accepted as an effective remedy for orchitis, spermatorrhea, and for cases of sexual impotence especially when caused by excesses. Some Mexican physicians also employ it as a brain tonic and for conditions of nervous debility and exhaustion.

Medical herbalists in different countries agree on the Mexican classification of damiana. In his monumental work, *Materia Medica Vegetablis*, Steinmetz of Holland cites damiana as follows:

"The leaves are a stimulant in sexual weakness and a tonic

to the nerves. The drug is esteemed for its aphrodisiac properties and its excellent effect on the reproductive organs. It overcomes exhaustion and cerebral lassitude, and a tendency in loss of power in the limbs. It is also diuretic."

In *Potter's Cyclopaedia of Botanical Drugs and Preparations* (England), we read:

"Damiana is very largely prescribed on account of its aphrodisiac qualities, and there is no doubt that it has a very great and generally beneficial action on the reproductive organs. It also acts as a tonic to the nervous system."

Early in the century, W. H. Meyers, an American physician, wrote:

"I have given it [damiana] quite an extensive trial in my practice and as a result I find that in cases of partial impotence or other sexual debility, its success is universal."

Damiana is used as a tea, or in the form of a fluid or dry extract. Professor Maximino Martinez of Mexico says, "An infusion of damiana is prepared with a teaspoon of leaves to a cup of water, taken before breakfast. Fifty drops of the extract in sweetened water or wine may also be taken daily.

AGNUS CASTUS

Botanical Name: *Vitex agnus castus*
Common Name: Chaste Tree

This beautiful plant is native to the shores of the Mediterranean. It was well known in early Egyptian and Arabian medicine as a priceless remedy for its healing influence on the sexual organism.

In modern times, the remedial value of Agnus castus is being rediscovered and it is rapidly gaining popularity in Germany, England, and other European nations. Medical herbalists consider it very beneficial for treating male disorders, especially premature old age from abuse of sexual power. It is given in symptoms of impotence, parts cold, relaxed, desire gone; scanty emission without ejaculation; loss of prostatic fluid on straining; testicles cold, swollen, hard, and painful.

Agnus castus is available in tablet form, with directions given on the bottle. In homeopathy, the tiny pellets prepared from the plant are used in doses of the first to sixth potency.

MELILOT

Botanical Name: *Melilotus officinalis*
Common Names: Honey Lotus, White Melilot, Yellow Melilot

The melilots are perennial herbs bearing sweet-scented white or yellow flowers. When the flowers are dried, the aroma becomes stronger, somewhat like that of the Tonka bean. One of the common names of the plant comes from the words *mel* (honey) and *lotus*, meaning honey lotus.

This plant can be found growing in many countries of the world, as it has great adaptability to a wide variety of climates and soils. It grows abundantly in the Yangtse provinces of China, and the Chinese use it as a medicine and burn it as an incense. In some lands the dried plant is used in making tobacco and snuff, or placed among linens to impart a pleasant fragrance. In Switzerland it is an ingredient of the green Swiss cheese called Schabzieger.

Remedial Uses

In herbal medicine, melilot is classed as aromatic, carminative, emollient, stimulant, and alterative. Taken as a tea it is said to be a helpful organ remedy for the penis, where there is weakness or lack of tone, and partial impotence. The herb is prepared like ordinary tea and one cup taken three times a day.

CHINESE SUPER OLD-FASHIONED COMPOUND HERB TEA

In the chapter on urinary disorders we cited this ancient Chinese herb formula and pointed out that along with treating urinary ailments it was also used by Chinese men for relieving or preventing prostate trouble. General directions for using the tea are the same, that is, the liquid contents of the preparation are poured into a container which is covered with a lid and heated until the tea is warm enough to drink. When the brew is heated, care is taken in removing the cover of the container so that the steamy droplets that form on the inside of the lid do not fall into the tea, as this would cause the beverage to lose some of its potency. The tea is taken on an empty stomach. Fruits and vegetables are not eaten for 48 hours after the tea is taken.

Additional Directions

For moderate or mild cases of prostate trouble, the Chinese Old-Fashioned Compound Herb Tea called *Fancy* is taken once a day until the condition has cleared up. The Chinese maintain that this tea is also a good preventative of prostate trouble if taken once a month or every other month.

For more stubborn prostate trouble, the stronger two-bottle set known as Super 1 and Super 2 compound tea is used. The bottle of Super 1 tea is heated and taken, followed three hours later by heating and drinking the bottle of Super 2 tea. It is said that generally this brings the desired results, but if necessary, another two-bottle set can be taken again the next day or for the next few days until definite results are achieved.

Case Histories

• Mr. J. H. writes: "I suffered from enlarged prostate gland, and had a terrible time straining to urinate which was very painful. After taking a set of special herb teas called Chinese Old-Fashioned Super 1 and 2, I was greatly relieved of pain, but still could not completely empty my bladder. So I took a second set of the Chinese Super teas, and ever since then I can urinate freely and completely, with no further trouble."

• Mr. W., age 52, complained of tenderness, throbbing, and pain in the region of the prostate gland, extending to the testicles. He writes: "My condition was diagnosed as enlarged prostate and orchitis. A friend of mine told me he had prostate trouble a year ago and was cured by taking Super 1 and 2 Chinese Old-Fashioned herb teas, so I decided to try them. After using the teas, I have had no further symptoms, and my doctor has given me a clean bill of health."

• A Chinese-American gentleman reported that during a vacation in Mexico he became very ill and suffered complete stoppage of urine. He writes: "A Mexican physician told me my prostate gland was badly swollen, and after catherizing me to get rid of the urine, he gave me a catheter to use until I could get back home to the States and see a urologist.

"I left for home immediately, but instead of seeing a urologist I went to a Chinese herbalist. He gave me two sets of Super 1 and Super 2 Chinese Old-Fashioned Compounded Herb Tea, which I drank on two consecutive days. At the end of that short time I could urinate freely without using the catheter tube. These good results were not temporary but lasting. Eighteen months have passed and I am still fine. I take one set of the two teas every two or three months as a preventative."

SUMMARY

1. There are a number of different ailments, for example, impotence, spermatorrhea, enlarged prostate, orchitis, and so on, that can affect the human male.

2. According to medical science, some difficulty with the prostate gland is a rather common occurence in men as they grow older.

3. One of the earliest signs of an ailing prostate is difficulty in urinating. If the prostate continues to enlarge, complete stoppage of urine may occur due to pressure of the gland upon the bladder. As a result, the accumulation of urine in the bladder may cause infection.

4. There are a number of herbal remedies from which to choose for coping with sexual inadequacies and other ailments that affect members of the male sex.

5. Many plants and herbs contain valuable ingredients that provide nutrition to the various sex glands and organs of the reproductive system.

6. The ancient formula known as Chinese Super Old-Fashioned Compounded Herb Tea is one of the most highly prized Chinese remedies for treating or preventing prostate trouble.

CHAPTER 11

Natural Remedies for Arthritis, Rheumatism, and Related Ailments

Mr. George Charles of Liverpool, England, was plagued with chronic arthritis for ten years, and the condition was worsening to the degree that he felt he would eventually become an invalid. After several weeks of drinking a tea prepared from an herb called Devil's Claw, he describes his improvement as amazing and says he feels like a new man.

In an interview in a British newspaper[1] he says:

"I must admit that I was very skeptical about the herb. After all, the doctors tried every conventional medicine on me, even steroids, and none of them had any effect. Some days the arthritis would really flare up and I would be unable to move at all. Then a friend told me of a plant called Devil's Claw which was used in Africa as a cure-all and which some German doctors were administering to people suffering from arthritis. Apparently they were achieving exciting cures. I decided I might as well try it."

Karen Brown, a nine-year-old school girl of England, suffered the terrible pain of rheumatoid arthritis from the age of

---

[1]*Liverpool Weekly News*, November 11, 1976.

five. Years of all types of orthodox medical treatment were of no avail, and finally the doctors declared that a remission of symptoms was hopeless.

Karen's teachers and classmates at St. Joseph's School took up a collection to send the child to Lourdes. Although the trip did not help Karen's condition in any way, her parents felt their prayers were answered almost a year later when their daughter began treatment with Devil's Claw. Karen's mother said: "This is the first time since Karen was struck down with rheumatoid arthritis that she has been able to play like an ordinary child." Karen now has a certificate in gymnastics and has also learned to swim.

Let us consider this remarkable plant, Devil's Claw, and a few of the many other natural remedies used in various countries of the world for the treatment of arthritis, rheumatism, and related ailments.

DEVIL'S CLAW

Botanical Name: *Harpagophytum procumbens*
Common Names: Grapple Plant, Kalahari, Skapkelu, Teufelskralle

This herb is found in the Nambian Steppes and the adjacent Kalahari Desert of South Africa. Its common name of Devil's Claw was given because of the thorny, barbed claws of the seed pod. The root prepared as a tea is highly valued by the Nambian natives who use it for a wide variety of ailments, including arthritis, rheumatism, and gout.

Medical Evidence

The majority of clinical tests with Devil's Claw root have been undertaken by German medical research teams. Professor Zorn of the University of Jena began experimental testing of the roots on lab animals, in which arthritis was induced. When inflammation reached its peak, treatment with Devil's Claw was begun. Prepared infusions of the herb were administered both by subcutaneous injections and orally by means of a tube down the throat.

Professor Zorn and his colleagues reported a definite lessening of swelling after the first injection. As treatment continued, the swelling was reduced progressively, and after five weeks it subsided and the joints were freely movable.

Dr. Zorn concludes:[2]

The infusion produces a pronounced diminution in swelling with full restoration in joint movement whether administered orally or subcutaneously. It is noteworthy that after treatment has been discontinued, the healing set in train continues. Lay opinion concerning the healing properties of Harpagophytum (Devil's Claw) root in rheumatic diseases can thus be accepted as true and is supported by our animal studies.

Dr. Sigmund Schmidt of Bad Rothenfelde has treated 200 rheumatic patients with Devil's Claw tea. He discovered that the tea had to be taken for an extended period of time before its beneficial effects were noted, depending on how severe the rheumatism was.

In addition to its favorable effects on conditions of rheumatism, Dr. Schmidt reports that Devil's Claw tea produced good results in certain disorders of the liver and kidneys. Most patients with liver and kidney ailments who were tested with the tea showed a return to normal within six weeks. Dr. Schmidt also considers Devil's Claw "an addition to our herbal armory against the poisoning of modern times," and adds that the herb "wonderfully stimulates the detoxicating and protective mechanisms of the body."[3]

Another German physician, Dr. von Korvin-Karsinski, an expert on East Asian and Indian medicine, found that Devil's Claw brought about improvement in rheumatic conditions and a variety of other ailments. He states that it has "extraordinary versatility as a therapeutic remedy," that it is a general strengthener of the glandular system, and has an "all-around cleansing effect on the organism."

In addition he says:

Quite apart from these wholly beneficial effects upon the kidney, bladder, gall and other organs, there is a general feeling of improved well-being. You could compare it with the good early morning feeling after a brief but deep sleep. Add the accompanying noticeable relief that climbing stairs is no longer an effort and you have an idea of the uplift you feel.[4]

Dr. Vogel, the well-known Swiss medical herbalist, traveled

---

[2]*Zeitschrift fur Rhemaforschung*, 1958.
[3]*Thereapiewoche*, 1972.
[4]*Die geistige Erde*, 1960.

to Southwest Africa to study Devil's Claw. He reports that the natives find the herb to be effective for kidney and liver ailments, and he states further:

> The tea will also ease complaints of rheumatism and gout. The natives of the seaport Swakomund in Nambia are exposed to these ailments especially during fall and winter months. What a blessing that this very helpful plant thrives nearby to be used as a most reliable remedy. Everybody states that nothing can be compared to the effectiveness of this tea of the desert. The cleansing and curing done within the body by this tea is proven in urine analysis done while under treatment. Such a test will show an astonishing discharge of uric acid, which is the cause of the ailments just mentioned.[5]

No Side Effects Noted

Aside from the fact that diabetics should not take Devil's Claw except under medical supervision, there seems to be as yet no known reason why anyone can not try the remedy.

Professor J. R. Mose of the Hygen Institute of Graz, Austria, reported testing the root for tolerance and finding no harmful side effects even after prolonged use.

Many other qualified medical experts have treated numerous human patients with Devil's Claw and are also convinced of the safety and reliability of the herb.

Clinical studies on the administration of Devil's Claw on lab animals have been done repeatedly in several different countries, yet there have been no unfavorable reactions of any kind even though extremely large quantities were administered.

In reference to the use of Devil's Claw, Dr. Vogel reports, "The tea is completely harmless and will not cause any side effects."

Methods of Using Devil's Claw

Devil's Claw root may be prepared as a tea, or taken in tablet form. The tea bag is placed in an enamel or Pyrex container and ¾ of a pint of boiling hot water is poured over it. The bag is allowed to remain in the container of water overnight and removed the next morning. The tea is taken in three equally divided doses ten minutes before each meal—breakfast, lunch

---

[5]*Gesundheitsnachrichten*, July 1973.

and dinner. Sugar must not be added to the tea as it has a negating effect on the herb's constituents.

If the tablets are used, one tablet is swallowed with a small glass of water three times daily, ten minutes before meals.

Generally, no real benefits are experienced from taking the tablets or tea for the first two or three weeks, but as the course of treatment continues, relief usually follows.

Most people have found it is best to use the tea or tablets for a course of eight or nine weeks. At the end of that period, Devil's Claw is discontinued for two or three weeks, then repeated again as needed.

> NOTE: Research teams have demonstrated that it is the secondary roots or tubers of the herb that produce effective amounts of the active ingredients, whereas the main root contains only minimal amounts. Therefore it is necessary to use only those products of Devil's Claw which state they are made solely from the secondary tubers or roots.

Case Histories

• "I thought I would try 'Devil's Claw.' At least it's natural. At first I didn't think it was doing any good, but during the third week I was amazed. My hands were back to normal. The ache went.

"I took a two-month course. I have had no trouble for six weeks. I still get slight pins and needles. The secret is not to break the two-month course of treatment. After the third week you will see and feel the difference." —Mrs. E. T.

• "Arthritis was starting in my knees, and my doctor told me it was something I'd have to live with, that he could not help me. I refused to accept this depressing view, so I went to an herbalist. The herbalist gave me Devil's Claw tablets to take, which have been a blessing. The stiffness and swelling in my knees is gone. I wonder how many other people with arthritis just accept the medical opinion that there is no help, and suffer in silence? If your doctor cannot help, take hope as I did and look elsewhere."—Mr. L.W.

• "For years I had been taking pain-killing medication for my arthritis. Then I heard about Devil's Claw tea. After two months of using the tea I find there has been much improvement as the pain is gone and I no longer need to take drugs. The tea also cured my indigestion." —Mrs. E. W.

NETTLE

Botanical Name: *Urtica dioica*
Common Names: Stinging Nettle, Common Nettle

In Germany, nettle is a favorite remedy for neuralgia. A decoction is prepared by simmering one and a half ounces of nettle in 12 ounces of water for ten or 15 minutes. When cool, it is strained, then reheated, and four tablespoons taken hot several times a day. In addition a poultice is prepared by placing a handful of nettles in a muslin bag and steeping in hot water for ten minutes. The poultice is applied, as hot as can be comfortably borne, to the painful area and repeated as necessary.

In some lands, nettle is also a favorite remedy for sciatica. Two ounces of nettles are simmered in one quart of water for 15 or 20 minutes. The decoction is allowed to stand until cool, then strained. It is then reheated and taken hot, one teacupful every two hours. As an accessory treatment, a second decoction of nettles is prepared in the same way, and used as hot fomentations which are applied locally to relieve the pain.

CHINESE TIGER BALM

Tiger Balm is a popular Oriental herb ointment developed more than half a century ago by two Chinese brothers. This fragrant herb product comes in two strengths, mild and strong.

Tiger balm is used as a soothing rub for the relief of minor pains of rheumatism and muscular aches and pains due to strains, fatigue, exposure or colds. For such conditions the affected parts are well rubbed with the Chinese herb ointment two or three times a day and covered with warm flannel.

GARLIC MILK

Garlic milk is considered an effective remedy for sciatica, by the Ayurvedic, Unani, and Tibbi systems of herbal medicine in India and Pakistan. It is also valued for the same purpose in many other countries. For example, Dr. Vogel of Switzerland writes:[6]

A garage mechanic who had suffered from sciatica for some considerable time, and for whom the doctor could do no more,

---

[6]*The Nature Doctor*, Bioforce-Verlag, Teufen (A R), Switzerland, 1959.

was advised to drink garlic milk daily. He took the advice, and within a few days the sciatica was greatly relieved. At the end of a fortnight the pain had completely disappeared.

Garlic milk may be prepared cooked or uncooked. Uncooked it has a more potent effect, but the cooking lessens the smell somewhat and the effect is still quite good. To prepare: crush the garlic, add it to the uncooked milk, or if you wish, the garlic may be cooked a little in the milk. To achieve a really intensive effect, you should drink about one-half pint of this mixture per day.

Of course, everyone does not react in the same way and not every remedy has the same effect on different people, but in cases of bad sciatica, it is worth giving this simple remedy a trial.

PECTIN

Pectin is a substance found in the cell walls of plants. Because of its ability to gel and hold water molecules together, pectin is valuable in ridding the body of toxins.

Certo is perhaps the best-known fruit pectin sold commercially on the market; however pectin is also available in tablet form.

As a domestic remedy for bursitis or tennis elbow, one tablespoonful of fruit pectin, such as Certo, is stirred in a small glass of water or fruit juice, and taken daily, or pectin tablets may be used. If you mix the pectin with fruit juice, use an alkaline juice such as apricot or apple.

CRUDE BLACKSTRAP MOLASSES

In reference to arthritis, J. W. Oliver of England writes:

"A most valuable food remedy is blackstrap molasses, one teaspoonful in three-fourths of a cup of hot water to be drunk before each meal, and in bad cases on rising and retiring each day. On this treatment alone arthritics have been able to discard their canes in a few weeks.

"Arthritis is more deepseated than rheumatism. It takes a long time 'coming on,' and can't be shaken off in twenty minutes. But perseverance along the lines indicated, however severe the case, will invariably score a victory in the end."

Other plant remedies reported to be effective in treating arthritis and rheumatism include chapparal, potato, cabbage, and alfalfa. (See *Magic Herbs for Arthritis, Rheumatism and Related Ailments,* Parker Publishing Company, Englewood Cliffs, N.J., 1981.)

SUMMARY

1. Devil's Claw Root is used as a natural remedy for various ailments, especially arthritis and rheumatism.

2. Generally no real benefits are experienced from taking Devil's Claw tablets or tea for the first two or three weeks, but as the course of treatment continues, relief usually follows.

3. For best results, Devil's Claw is taken for a course of eight or nine weeks. At the end of that period the remedy is discontinued for two or three weeks, then resumed again as needed.

4. Medical teams who have tested Devil's Claw reported there were no side effects from its use. However, diabetics should not use the herb except under medical supervision.

5. There are a number of other natural remedies that have a beneficial effect on some cases of arthritis, rheumatism, and related ailments.

CHAPTER 12

Propolis—Nature's Miracle Healing Substance

Propolis is a sticky resinous substance collected by bees from the bark or leaf buds of trees, especially poplars which are the most important source. Its medicinal value has been known since ancient times. In the first century A.D., Celsus, the Roman philosopher, wrote instructions on preparing resin poultices with propolis. Pliny, whose writings consisted of 37 volumes of which seven were devoted to medical botany, suggested a mixture of barley flour and propolis as a treatment for abcesses. Dioscorides, a physician to the Roman army in Asia during the first century A.D., wrote of the healing virtues of propolis. This remarkable substance was also cited in the Persian, Arabic and Koran manuscripts of the 6th and 8th centuries as an effective remedy for bronchial catarrhs, blood purification, and skin disorders.

In later centuries, Gerard, Culpeper, and other early British medical herbalists also cited propolis in their writings.

Today, interest in this natural healing substance has been revived, and its effectiveness in treating a variety of ailments is being scientifically proven in many parts of the world.

Constituents in Propolis

Soviet medical research teams have analyzed propolis and reported that it contains resin, balsam, wax, fragrant essential oils, pollen, organic and amino acids. It is rich in minerals, antibiotics and vitamins, especially the B vitamins, and also contains phytoncides, tannic acid, and other ingredients.

A Remedy for Many Ills

• Scientist K. Lund Aagaard of Denmark spent 20 years researching the medicinal value of propolis. He reported that tests on over 50,000 volunteers proved that the substance totally or partly cures bacterial and viral infections of the intestines, eyes, mouth, throat, nose, stomach complaints and numerous skin diseases.

• Dr. Rudolph Rey of Kornenburg, Germany, says that propolis helps against poor blood circulation, migraine headaches, and dizziness.

• Doctors at the Klosterneuburg Hospital in Austria used propolis for treating 250 patients suffering from ailments ranging from stomach ulcers to colitis and severe gastric conditions. Two hundred and forty-four were reportedly healed within two weeks. In one study, Dr. Franz K. Feiks reported that a group of patients suffering from stomach ulcers were given three drops of propolis before meals, three times daily. In seven out of ten cases, pain had disappeared within three days. After ten days, no wounds could be detected in six out of ten patients.

• Dr. Edith Lauda of Austria tested propolis for its antibacterial effect on the human skin. Sixty patients who had been suffering for several years with acne were treated with propolis tincture and propolis ointments. Twenty-five cases of acne *simplex* were completely healed at home within seven days. Thirty-five cases of a more difficult form of acne were healed in three weeks. In addition to home treatment, these cases had only three weekly treatments at the clinic.

One patient had been treated for 30 years for *acne conglobata* by a large number of dermatologists with no results. After only two treatments with propolis, her skin was free of inflammation, and only very small marks of acne remained visible.

Another spectacular case was that of a patient, aged 40, who had *acne pustulosa* which covered her whole face. Orthodox therapy had not helped, yet within two weeks of home treatment with propolis ointment and tincture, the acne had completely disappeared.

• At a symposium in Yugoslavia, Dr. Franz Feiks reported that he treated 21 cases of shingles by applying propolis tincture as a dressing to the affected parts. In 48 hours pain had disappeared in all 21 cases and did not recur. The skin sores in 19 of the patients were completely healed.

• In Russia, cases of neurodermatitis and dry eczema reportedly have been cured by applying a propolis ointment twice daily. It was pointed out, however, that the ointment was not effective for wet eczemas. In such cases, the ointment aggravated the conditions.

• Soviet literature reports that some types of hearing defects have been successfully treated with an alcoholic tincture of propolis mixed with olive or corn oil. Patients were treated by placing into the ear a wad of gauze saturated with the propolis mixture. For adult cases, the gauze plug was left for 36 to 38 hours and the treatment repeated 10 or 12 times. Three hundred and fourteen out of 382 patients treated experienced improved hearing, and some patients reported considerable relief from head noises.

• Dr. R. Chauvin of Paris, France, says he has found that the use of propolis can help prevent viral infections such as flu, colds, and tonsillitis.

• Professor Osmanagic of Yugoslavia tested 270 volunteers who were exposed to influenza. Eighty-eight took propolis, and 182 did not. Of the group who used propolis, only 7% caught the flu, while 63% of the group who had not taken the substance contracted the flu.

• Very good results from the use of propolis on patients with inflammation of the mucous membranes of the throat and mouth were reported by Professor Kern of the Ear, Nose, and Throat Clinic at Ljubljana, Yugoslavia. The patients dissolved a propolis lozenge in the mouth every two hours, Within six to ten hours after starting the treatment, almost all patients were free of fever and swallowing was painless.

In cases of patients suffering from chronic inflammation of the mouth and gums, symptoms were scarcely noticeable by the next day. In some instances, especially of children, improvement had taken place within only a few hours.

Another ear, nose, and throat specialist of Yugoslavia prescribed tincture of propolis on small cubes of sugar which could be sucked, for a four-year-old girl suffering from severe tonsillitis. After two doses her temperature had dropped and her appetite returned. Subsequent examination by the specialist showed the tonsils to be clear and free of inflammation.

• Dr. M. M. Frenkel of Russia found propolis to be effective in treating diseases of the sinuses and upper part of the respiratory tract.

• Some doctors in America are starting to study propolis. Dr. Roy Kupsinel of Florida prescribed propolis for many of his patients and has found that when the substance is taken regularly it creates an antibiotic disease-fighting reaction to almost any illness, without side effect. Dr. John Diamond of Texas considers propolis a powerful substance for stimulating the thymus gland, thereby strengthening the body's immune system.

• Propolis has been used in various countries for treating cuts, bruises, burns, corns, warts, toothache, radiation sickness, and infections of the bladder, kidney, prostate gland, and sexual organs.

Preparations of Propolis

Propolis comes in many forms, e.g., capsules containing finely ground propolis in a gelatin base, lozenges, tooth paste, propolis skin cream, and Savaskin Propolis which is a tincture and can be used as an overall skin tonic, or for various ailments. Such preparations are available from herb firms and health food stores.

How Propolis May Be Used

Respiratory Ailments: Propolis is helpful as a soothing agent.

• For coughs and colds a propolis lozenge is sucked as often as needed.
• For tonsillitis, the lozenge is used three or four times daily.
• In conditions of sore throat, a propolis lozenge is taken every hour until relief is obtained. Gargling with four or five drops of Salvaskin propolis tincture in a small glass of warm water is soothing to a sore throat. For sinusitis, a propolis lozenge is chewed as often as required.
• To prevent the common cold, one teaspoon of propolis

diluted with honey is taken daily for 40 to 50 consecutive days during the cold season.

Gum Disorders: Propolis toothpaste is used as a regular toothpaste for treating or preventing gum disorders. In addition, for gum disorders, one propolis lozenge is chewed three or four times a day.

Dry Eczema: Propolis skin cream is applied once daily, and for the first three or four days of the treatment, one propolis capsule is taken twice daily.

Psoriasis: The same instructions as those given for eczema are followed for psoriasis.

Warts: Propolis tincture is dabbed on the wart once or twice daily.

Shingles: Propolis skin cream is applied at night before retiring. In addition, one propolis capsule is taken twice a day, between meals.

Ulcers: For stomach and intestinal ulcers, one propolis capsule is taken three times daily, one-half hour before meals.

Bruises, Cuts, Blemishes: Propolis is combined with honey and applied to the area with gauze. The bandage is allowed to remain overnight, and replaced daily until healed.

Burns: Applying a few drops of propolis to a burn reportedly gives relief and speeds healing.

Abcess: Salvaskin tincture of propolis is applied to the affected part.

Cystitis: Cystitis and other urinary conditions have been improved by taking one propolis capsule three times daily.

Prostate Trouble: One capsule of propolis is taken three times daily.

Migraine Headache: For migraine headache, one propolis capsule is taken twice a day.

NOTE: Although propolis is a natural substance which can be of considerable benefit, tests at the Department of Dermatology, Royal Infirmary, Edinburgh, Scotland, showed that a few people (approximately only one person in every two thousand) are sensitive to propolis. Anyone who develops a rash after taking the substance either orally or externally, should stop the treatment. The rash reportedly disappears as soon as the propolis treatment has been discontinued.

SUMMARY

1. Propolis is a sweet-smelling resinous substance collected by bees from the bark and leaf buds of various trees, especially poplars.
2. Propolis has been known and used as a folk remedy since ancient times.
3. Today, propolis is being rediscovered by researchers into natural medicine.
4. Doctors and medical teams from many parts of the world are proving that propolis is an effective remedy for a variety of ailments.
5. Scientists have analyzed propolis and found that it contains natural antibiotics, valuable nutrients, and other ingredients.
6. Propolis is available in various forms, and these preparations can be obtained from herb firms and health food stores.

CHAPTER 13

Eleuthero—Nature's Wonder Herb

With colossal research facilities to speed them on, Soviet scientists have been very successful in their continued search for old, new, or rare plants that contain properties useful in modern medicine. One startling breakthrough was the discovery that Asiatic ginseng, a plant used for thousands of years in Chinese folk medicine, is a treasure house of valuable therapeutic powers. Another important finding was that pectin, a substance derived from sunflower seeds, provides a built-in protection against accumulation of radioactive matter in the human system.

Now a new miracle of nature has been discovered and acclaimed by Soviet scientists. This is a plant known botanically as *Eleutherococcus senticosus*. It is a tall shrub native to southern regions of the Soviet Far East, belonging to the same Araliaceae family as Panax ginseng. The flowers of the eleutherococcus bush are yellowish or violet, and the leaves similar in appearance to those of ginseng. Nikolay Suprunov, a young Soviet scientist, observed that spotted deer hungrily devoured the leaves of eleutherococcus. The shrub blooms in July, and bears clusters of dark purple berry-like fruits which ripen in September. Because its branches are spiked with thorns, people in olden times named the plant "Touch-me-not" and "Devil's Bush," and these synonyms are still in use today. More modern names for eleutherococcus are

"Siberian ginseng," or simply "Eleuthero" (pronounced El-oó-ther-oh) for short.

RUSSIAN SCIENTIFIC STUDIES ON ELEUTHERO

The eleuthero plant has been given extensive scientific testing by Drs. I. I. Brekhman, Z. I. Gutnikova, P. V. Vorobyeva, N. I. Suprunov, and other researchers at the Far Eastern Center of the Siberian Division of the USSR Academy of Science. Results have established that a fluid extract of eleuthero possesses a remarkably wide range of therapeutic activity. For example, it protects the body against stress, radiation, and various chemical toxins; reduces elevated sugar content in the blood; has a beneficial effect in functional nervous disorders; normalizes low blood pressure and mild forms of high blood pressure; produces a therapeutic effect in the initial stages of atherosclerosis; reduces high cholesterol levels in the blood. As a tonic, it relieves brain fag, gives more mental alertness and better coordination of bodily functions; restores loss of vigor and vitality; increases endurance; improves vision and hearing acuity; produces a strengthening effect in convalescence after serious illness or surgery, and in exhaustion and debility due to chronic illness.

Let us discuss these and the many other therapeutic effects of eleuthero in more detail.

ELEUTHERO—A FIRST-CLASS ADAPTOGEN

The term "adaptogen" has been used in Soviet medical writings in recent years, and has also appeared in Anglo-American medical literature. In order to be classified as an adaptogen, a substance must meet the following qualifications:

1. It must be non-toxic, or at least toxicity must be extremely low.
2. Its action should be nonspecific; that is, it should increase resistance to a wide variety of adverse influences, physical, chemical, and biological in nature—e.g., stress, overexertion, various toxins, infection by some contagious agents.
3. It should possess a normalizing action—for example, a tendency to normalize high or low blood pressure, underactive or overactive glands, low or high blood sugar, etc.

According to published reports in Soviet medical journals,

eleutherococcus meets all the requirements necessary to be classified as an adaptogen. The Russians state that "side effects due to eleutherococcus are very rare." These effects include slight drowsiness immediately after taking a dose of eleuthero extract on an empty stomach, or short-term sleep disturbances if the extract is taken directly before bedtime. These side effects are stated to be easily remedied by taking the extract after meals, and not at bedtime. Only a relatively few persons experienced the side effects.

The Most Reliable of All Adaptogens Known

As an adaptogen, the Soviets place eleutherococcus first, followed by Panax ginseng. As in the case of ginseng, eleuthero produces a stimulant effect when taken in a single dose, and a tonic effect when taken in repeated doses over a more or less long period of time. Dr. Brekhman says that eleuthero is "the most reliable and efficaceous of all adaptogenic agents presently known." He adds, "It is absolutely safe, has a broad range of therapeutic action, does not cause shifts in normal physiological functions of the organism, normalizes pathological shifted functions, increases the organism's resistance to adverse factors of physical, chemical, and biological nature."

Eleuthero Experiments on Farm Animals

Tests with eleutherococcus on farm animals produced startling results. Cows gave more milk, chicks became full grown hens in two months, and bees increased their production of honey by 30 to 60 percent. Experiments with minks revealed that eleuthero reduced sterility and diminished by 50% the number of stillborn cubs. The animals' pedigree qualities also improved.

Rabbits, swine, horses, deer, and dogs were administered eleuthero for a period ranging from a few days to a year. In all these experiments, the plant extract invariably produced only favorable results.

Experiments on Lab Animals

Other tests conducted on lab animals revealed that a liquid extract of eleutherococcus *roots* increased work endurance by 25%; a preparation of the *leaves* by 44%; and a mixture of both *roots* and *leaves* by a full 70 percent!

Tests on Humans Favorable

Later, under clinical conditions, the adaptogenic effect of eleuthero was studied on humans. It was established that the plant extract increased physical endurance and mental efficiency. This was attended by other favorable effects, such as general improvement in health and spirits (better appetite and sleep; absence of moodiness, anxiety, and depression, etc.). It was also noted that eleuthero strengthens the visual acuity, and if taken over a long period of time, also improves the auditory acuity.

Work Capacity Improved

As with ginseng, the stimulant and tonic action of eleuthero was tested on telegraph operators. It is recognized that this type of work requires deep concentration, quick reaction, extract coordination of movements, and great physical endurance.

It was found that the plant extract remarkably improved the work performance of the operators. There was finer coordination of mental and physical reflexes, stamina and endurance were increased, better concentration was noted (for example, the number of mistakes the operators generally made was reduced).

Eleutherococcus extract was also tested at the Lesgraft Institute of Physical Culture and Sports. The extract delivered a positive invigorating effect on sportsmen engaged in various sports activities. The athletes noted an increase of vitality and endurance, significant improvement of reflex action, and better concentration.

Such improvements in reaction times to various stimuli are of even greater importance when you consider them in relation to health hazards. The ability to react faster in a crisis is of major concern—for instance in the split second before an automobile accident, when the ability to react quicker could often avert collision, prevent serious injuries or fatalities.

A WIDE RANGE OF APPLICATION

According to Soviet researchers, the adaptogenic action of eleuthero is of value in illness as it increases bodily resistance. It is also a helpful restorative in cases of debility and emaciation which accompany chronic ailments, and for convalescence after surgery or after a bout of illness. In addition, Dr. Brekhman reports that the action of eleuthero "permits one to use it not only for various pathological conditions but also for healthy persons in cases of overfatigue or necessity to work in difficult condition unfavorable for the organism. In such cases, eleutherococcus is an excellent therapeutic for restoring the working capacity, as well as prophylactic [preventative or protective agent] which can be used in view of hard work, or in cases of instability and sharp changes in the weather. In the latter case, the prophylactic use of eleutherococcus results in a reduction of general morbidity and the rate of infections in particular."

Protection Against Temperature Extremes

Working in extreme heat, such as mowing a lawn on a very hot day, or working in bitter cold weather (for example, shoveling snow in freezing temperatures), strains the body and is especially hazardous to people with heart or circulatory problems. Winter is not only unpleasant, but in general seems to encourage illness such as colds and many other infections.

Experimenting with lab animals, Soviet scientists found that overheating of white mice causes the rodents' death. But when mice were given eleuthero, a protective effect was noted as the thermal endurance of the mice increased. Cooling the animals down to 17° or 16°C for only two minutes caused detrimental shifts in their physiological functions, but "even a single dose of eleutherococcus diminishes the intensity of these pathological changes."

An Aid Against Various Toxic Chemicals

The favorable antitoxic effects of eleuthero in cases of some infections, autointoxication, various toxic chemicals, alcohol, and some narcotic agents have been noted by Russian researchers. For example, mice were intoxicated with tetraethyl lead. When conditioned reflexes became damaged because of intoxication, half of the mice were treated with eleuthero. The treatment restored conditioned reflexes and prolonged the mice's lives. Untreated mice lived an average of 30 days; the treated mice, 40 days.

Of Value in Autointoxication

Autointoxication results from faulty elimination of the body's own toxic wastes. For instance, the putrefaction of decaying fecal wastes present in the intestines and clinging to the intestinal walls is absorbed into the blood stream. The body becomes polluted and the result is ill health. Professor Metchnikoff claimed that autointoxication is also a contributing factor to premature aging.

A Case History

One woman suffered for years with chronic autointoxication. The whites of her eyes had a dull gray cast. She had very little strength or energy, and felt only "half alive." She said that her existence was one continuous round of laxatives, enemas and colonics, which seemed to tax what little strength she had. Although these methods helped to eliminate some of the waste products from her body, they did not entirely remove the autointoxication.

The woman took a one-month course of eleuthero extract, and to her amazement noted that for the first time in years her eyes became clearer, and her strength increased. Following the directions for the use of eleuthero, she stopped taking the extract for one week, then immediately started another one-month course of the preparation. At the end of that time she reported that all of her symptoms of autotoxication had disappeared.

Helps Blood Donors

After donating a pint of blood, Soviet donors were given daily administrations of eleutherococcus extract. This resulted in restoration of the blood hemoglobin level within 13 days, whereas in ordinary cases (without eleuthero) it took a month to restore the level.

Benefits of Eleuthero in Atherosclerosis

Clinical studies of the therapeutic effect of eleuthero extract on atherosclerosis were undertaken by Dr. A. P. Golikov in Leningrad. In most patients, the condition involved mainly the coronary vessels and the aorta (large artery of the heart). In some patients the condition was complicated by hypertensive vascular diseases. Patients complained of weakness, exhaustion, pains in the heart, and pains beneath the breast bone. Most had increased cholesterol serum levels, and also showed signs of cardiac insufficiency.

Each patient was given a thorough examination, and then placed on a course of eleuthero treatment, one dose of 25 to 30 drops of the extract three times daily. The course lasted for 25 to 30 days. Of other medication, only nitroglycerine and validol were given when necessary. These particular patients remained on the job while undergoing the eleuthero treatment.

After only one week from the start of the eleuthero treatment, and especially after one month, the patients improved significantly. Weakness and exhaustion vanished, cardiac pains and headaches became less severe or disappeared entirely, especially in patients with normal or low blood pressure. Along with these therapeutic results, the eleuthero treatment was accompanied by an improvement of circulation, normalization of blood pressure, reduction of cholesterol levels, and favorable shifts in protein and lipid metabolism.

The positive effects lasted for two to four months after the first course of eleuthero treatment. Three to four months later, subsequent courses of the plant extract produced an even more stable improvement of the patients' general state.

During four years, some patients received six to eight courses of eleuthro treatment, without any additional medicines. In all cases, results were reported to be good. Commenting on this, Dr. Brekhman says: "Thus if favorable shifts in the organism can be produced by eleutherococcus alone, without additional therapeutic measures, one may assume that the use of this preparation in combination with specific antisclerotic medicines may be still more effective."

ACNE

Acne is a troublesome skin disease that especially embarrasses adolescents. Although this skin disorder is not dangerous to life, it can have serious consequences as it may cause personality disturbances or acute emotional upsets. There are instances where adolescents troubled by acne have become shy, introverted, bitter, irritable, or despondent. And the British *Journal of Dermatology* offers the opinion that there is a definite relationship between "the more disfiguring dermatoses such as acne" and antisocial behavior.

Acne usually disappears with advancing age, but unfortunately it often leaves pockmarks that can seem tragic to the victim.

Under the circumstances it should be of great interest to acne sufferers to learn that in some cases, eleuthero extract has proved to be an effective treatment and preventative of this skin disorder. For example:

• John C., a young high school student, noticed signs of acne appearing on his face. As the weeks passed the acne condition became more pronounced. In desperation he began squeezing the pimples, which only made matters worse. Normally a friendly, talkative, outgoing boy, John became a loner. His parents took him to several different medics, and found the treatments disappointing. A friend of the family, who had heard of eleuthero, suggested they have their son give it a try. After taking 25 drops in a little water, three times daily for a week, John noted a slight improvement in his condition. He continued the doses for another three weeks and was overjoyed to see that the acne was definitely clearing up. After another one-month course of the eleuthero extract, all signs of the skin disorder had disappeared.

• Bonny G., a popular high school cheerleader, became upset when she sighted an ugly pimple on her chin. But when more pimples began appearing on other areas of her face, she became almost hysterical. Bonny immediately resigned as cheerleader, in spite of the urging of her friends to reconsider. Dating, parties, and other social events were also out of the question as far as Bonny was concerned.

The young girl consulted many different medics, and many different treatments were tried. None were successful. One physician assured her that she would most likely outgrow the acne condition, which comforted Bonny not at all.

Eventually, the young cheerleader learned of eleuthero extract and heard that it had proved helpful in some cases of acne. She said, "I really didn't believe anything in the world could possibly help, so you can imagine my surprise when after taking three courses of eleuthero extract there was no longer a single trace of my miserable acne condition, and no pockmarks!"

DIABETES

Russian scientists report that experiments with animals have established that eleutherococcus, while not affecting the normal content of sugar in the blood, lowered this content if there was an alimentary or adrenalin hyperglycemia.

Dr. Brekhman writes: "In the laboratory of Professor K. A. Meshcherskaya, the effect of eleutherococcus on the course of a severe form of experimental [alloxan-induced] diabetes was studied. The administration of liquid eleutherococcus extract to rats twice a day resulted in a drop of urine sugar level by half, a diminution of weight loss of sick animals and doubling of their length of life.

"In cases of less severe form of diabetes the therapeutic effect was even more pronounced. The large amount of sugar excreted with the urine diminished three times; the total daily urine excretion and the blood sugar level decreased while the length of the rats' lives increased.

Clinical Studies of Diabetes in Humans

"The results of experimental therapeutic studies of eleutherococcus effect in the treatment of alloxan-induced diabetes in animals as well as some clinical observation give prospects to broad clinical studies of eleutherococcus in the treatment of diabetes. In patients suffering from light and moderate-gravity diabetes, the use of eleutherococcus extract in a dose of 40 drops three times daily resulted in a reduction of the blood sugar level by 15 to 25 mg%. In some cases the positive shifts were still more pronounced. For example, in patient Z (female) who had received a one-month course of eleutherococcus treatment, the blood sugar level fell from 140 mg%, and the urine sugar decreased gradually from 4 percent first, down to 3, then to 1, and at the end of the treatment down to 0.5 percent. Most patients showed a considerable improvement of their general state, weakness and fatigue became less pronounced, thirst and itching troubled them to a much lesser extent."

ELEUTHERO—NATURE'S ANSWER TO STRESS

Stressing challenges are as varied as life itself, and in today's modern world we have less and less opportunity to return to a relaxed state before another stress situation appears. The burden of continued stress, or intense sudden fright, can cause a breakdown of essential glands and organs. Unrelenting stress of frustration or suppression of anger is a frequent cause of headache. A few of the many other ailments cited by science that often arise from stress are ulcerative colitis, stomach ulcers, diabetes, respiratory infections, irritable colon, high blood pressure, and various skin disorders.

Some Interesting Cases

Many people have also claimed excellent results with the use of eleuthero in stress conditions. Here are some examples:

• A top executive suffered tension problems, and was in a highly agitated state. Insomnia, indigestion, and constipation plagued him. After she took eleuthero extract for two weeks he felt much better, his nagging symptoms lessened, and he was getting a good night's sleep. He continued taking the plant extract for another two weeks and claimed he was restored to a trouble-free condition.

• Mrs. G. F., married for 12 years, developed blinding headaches right after her husband suddenly announced that he wanted a divorce. Mrs. F. suffered periodically from these distressing headaches for six months. After taking a course of eleuthero extract, the head pains vanished, and there has been no recurrence for close to a year.

ELEUTHERO—NATURE'S NERVE TONIC

Among other factors, your ability to meet stress depends on strong, healthy nerves. Probing further into the secrets of eleuthero, Soviet experts discovered that the plant extract had a pronounced therapeutic effect on functional nervous disorders, even in chronic patients who had been previously treated by a variety of different medications which had not helped.

Clinical studies with the plant extract were carried out on patients suffering from nervous exhaustion, or nervous and emotional disturbances (not insanity). Their symptoms ranged from hair-trigger irritability, to moodiness, lethargy, apprehension, menopausal "blues," anxiety, feelings of impending doom, fears of heart trouble or insanity, persistent insomnia, depression, loss of vigor, and chronic fatigue.

In most patients, the administration of eleuthro extract brought about an improvement in sleep, restoration of energy and strength, a marked sense of well-being, and stimulated interest in life and work. The extract also displayed its normalizing effects in many areas. For example, while relieving symptoms of weakness, exhaustion, moodiness, and depression in patients suffering from these conditions, it produced on emotionally excited patients a calm, restful, and well-balanced effect.

Along with the corrective action in nervous conditions,

eleuthero also demonstrated its normalizing effect by reducing a high cholesterol level and increasing a low hemoglobin level in many patients. In cases of moderate leukopenia (lower than normal white cells circulating in the blood), the count was increased to normal, and in patients with leucocytosis (abnormally high number of white cells) the count was reduced to the proper level.

How Eleuthero Was Administered

The eleuthero treatment in these cases of nervous exhaustion, and nervous and emotional disturbances, lasted for four to five weeks. One dose of 20 to 40 drops of the extract was taken three times a day. To achieve a stable therapeutic effect, Dr. Brekhman says, "It is recommended to give two or three courses at one- or two-week intervals."

Note: A "course" means one month or five weeks of daily doses of eleuthero extract. At the end of that time, the doses are discontinued for one or two weeks, and then another course of eleuthero is taken.

Case Histories Involving Menopausal "Nerves"

The added stresses of physical changes normal to the menopause are reflected by the nervous system. One woman may find she is listless, depressed; another jumps at sudden noises or a mere tap on the shoulder; still another has her bad days in which she is irritable, short-tempered, dissatisfied with herself, her family, and her surroundings.

Eleuthero extract has proved highly beneficial in such conditions. For example:

• Mrs. J. R. had the menopausal blues which she said made it difficult to live with herself or anyone else. Normally an energetic happy woman, she became moody, depressed, tired, had fits of crying spells, and wanted nothing more than to be left alone.

• Mrs. R's sister-in-law was also experiencing menopausal difficulties, but by contrast she was tense, irritable, jittery, impatient, and quarrelsome.

The normalizing and tonic action of eleuthero worked wonders for both women. Mrs. R. experienced a stimulating effect that put zest and energy into her life, and her sister-in-law obtained a calm, soothing effect. The husbands of both women said they were delighted to have their wives "back again."

Case Histories Involving Other Functional Nervous Disorders

• Mrs. V. S. secured a challenging and responsible position with a growing business firm. As the months passed, she became nervous, agitated, and jittery, and suffered from heartburn, sour belchings, and nausea. She said, "Although I love my job, I go overboard and worry like the devil."

The young woman took a course of eleuthero, and found it to be a soothing and therapeutic nerve tonic. In a few weeks her distressing nervous symptoms began to subside, her stomach became more settled, and the heartburn less troublesome. She repeated the treatment and was delighted with her marked improvement. Her co-workers agreed that she had indeed because a relaxed, poised, and confident woman.

• Mr. C. L. told his friends: "Whenever I'm in a financial bind or have an argument with anyone—in fact when there is anything emotionally disturbing—I really get uptight, and have to take a pill in order to sleep. No matter how hard I try to keep my cool, the jangled nerves always bug me. One night when I was pacing the floor like a caged animal, my wife shoved two bottles of eleuthero at me. 'I bought these today, so for Pete's sake, try them,' she said. I did use them for several weeks, and found that he stuff really works! I've been feeling just great and haven't had a sleeping pill in four months."

HIGH AND LOW BLOOD PRESSURE

Hypertension (High Blood Pressure)

The usual symptoms of high blood pressure are dizziness, headaches, and noises or ringing in the ears.

Blood pressure means the force of the blood against the walls of the arteries. When the pressure is abnormally high, it naturally causes abnormal wear and tear on the blood vessels. In severe cases, the pressure can cause the strained capillaries (tiny blood vessels) to rupture, and result in a heart attack or stroke (cerebral hemorrhage). Stroke is the third leading cause of death in the United States.

The brain is believed to be particularly susceptible to hemorrages because it is enclosed in the skull and cannot expand when the blood pressure increases.

Hypotension (Low Blood Pressure)

In conditions of hypotension, the push or force of the blood against the vessel walls decreases, and the cells fail to receive an adequate supply of nutrients carried by the blood. Fatigue, sensitivity to cold and heat, rapid pulse beat on exertion, and lack of endurance, are the usual symptoms of low blood pressure. A person with this condition requires more sleep than a healthy individual, and generally finds himself more tired when he awakens in the morning than when he went to bed.

EFFECTS OF ELEUTHERO ON THE BLOOD PRESSURE

Results of carefully controlled studies by Soviet scientists have established the fact that eleuthero extract has a normalizing effect on the blood pressure. Dr. Brekhman writes: "It is known that eleutherococcus is one of the best remedies for curing hypotension [low blood pressure] but at the same time it reduces the elevated blood pressure in many hypertensive patients, or, in other words, displays its normalizing adaptogenic action." He points out that in conditions of high blood pressure, the reduction is gradual and moderate, except with those suffering from severe forms of high blood pressure, in which case the extract is not effective.

The extract does not disturb normal blood pressure.

ELEUTHERO PROTECTS AGAINST RADIATION DAMAGE

Roetgenotherapy (radiation treatment) is one of the life-saving methods used by medical science in the treatment of cancer. Unfortunately, however, there is always the risk of radiation injuries or radiation sickness which can cause severe complications in the patient's body. Some examples of the damaging effects that can occur after therapy with radioactive cobalt are radiation burns, hemorrhaging, severe anemia, dizziness, nausea, vomiting, and headaches.

Soviet scientists have established that eleutherococcus extract has a protective effect against radiation, and a therapeutic effect in acute and chronic radiation sickness. Experimenting first with animals, it was found that in a single X-ray irradiation of rats, eleuthero was shown to "possess medicinal and radioprotective action." In doses of 1620 and 7000 Rs in prolonged irradiation, eleuthero "doubled the life-time of rats, improved the state of blood and other indices."

Radioprotective Effect of Eleuthero on Humans

Eleutherococcus extract was used by Dr. T. M. Khatiashvili (Chair of Oncology of the Tbilisi Post-Graduate Medical School) in a complex therapy of lip and oral cancer. Two groups of 38 patients each were chosen, each group having cancerous tumors similar in character, stage of growth, and localization (lower lips, both lips, oral cavity).

One group of patients, ranging from 30 to 60 years of age, received a daily dose of eleuthero extract for 14 days. The preparation was taken by each of these patients one hour before a roentgenotherapy procedure. It was reported that "eleutherococcus considerably improved the patient's general state, appetite and sleep, and normalized pathological shifts of respiration, pulse and arterial pressure."

Both groups required approximately equal doses of radiation; however, in the group treated with eleuthero, tumors began to soften three to five days earlier, and the wound healed within four weeks instead of the usual one and a half to two months.

The patients of both groups remained under observation for two years. During this time, four patients of the control group (those not receiving eleuthero) developed relapses, and three developed metastases (the spread of cancer from its original site). In the same number of patients treated with eleuthero, neither relapses nor metastases occurred.

Additional Studies

The effect of eleutherococcus in combined therapy of mammary gland cancer was studied by specialists of the Institute of Oncology, the Ministry of Health of the Georgian SSR. Of these studies, Dr. Brekhman writes:

"There were eighty patients from 27 to 73 years of age with the diagnoses of mammary cancer of the first, second, and third degree. The patients were treated with ThioTEPA and deep roentgenotherapy. Half of them received eleutherococcus extract in a dose of 2 ml daily for 14 days. The patients had had radical or subradical operations. For each experimental group, about the same number of patients with tumors similar in form or stage were chosen for controls; the control patients received the same treatment, except for the administration of eleutherococcus. The most favorable results were observed when eleutherococcus was administered two to four days prior to the beginning of roentgenotherapy or in parallel with the latter. These patients showed almost no usual reactions to X-radiation, such as indisposition, dizziness, nausea, loss of appetite, etc. Their feelings of well-being and their general state remained good for a long time. Even in patients with third stage cancer whose state was grave, an improvement of mood, general state, and appetite could be achieved after taking three or four doses of eleutherococcus. The arterial pressure, pulse, and respiration rate in eleutherococcus-treated patients were much better than in control patients observed in parallel. No side effects were noted in any case."

Other Sources of Radiation Hazards

The discovery that eleutherococcus extract has a protective effect against radiation is extremely important, not only to patients receiving roentgenotherapy, but to all of us. A great many surveys conducted by scientists in the United States and elsewhere have indicated that the most damning cause responsible for most leukemias and bone cancers is radiation. Radiation does not only mean fallout from nuclear blasts, it also means X-rays, whether we get them from a surgeon, a general practitioner, a dentist, or an osteopath. If used wisely, and with caution, X-rays can be great life savers, but they can do much harm if used indiscriminately, as for example, having an X-ray when there's no reason to suspect a dental problem, or having a routine X-ray examination just to get a clean bill of health, unless there is reason to suspect ill health.

According to A. V. Topchiev, a Soviet researcher, everyone in the world already has dangerous amounts of radioactive strontium 90 in his or her bones. This has resulted from nuclear bomb tests of all kinds by the United States, Russia, China, and other nations. Dr. Topchiev predicts that within the foreseeable future there will be upwards of 200,000 cases of leukemia (blood cancer) from world-wide radioactive fallout alone.

AGING

According to a theory that is gaining general acceptance, aging is the result of destructive reactions caused by "free radicals" over a long period of time. Even a small amount of these free radicals can be damaging.

A free radical is a fragment of a molecule that has been torn away from its source and tends to join the body's normal molecules, which it can seriously damage, or even cause a chain reaction of molecular destruction. Cells die, enzymes fail to function, energy is reduced, and the body's ability to renew itself and resist and recover from illness is diminished.

It has been discovered that the destructive reactions caused by free radicals can be almost completely suppressed by what are called "antioxidants." In their experiments, scientists have prolonged life by using antioxidants to reduce the number of free radicals formed by oxidation.

As the result of extensive and complex studies, Soviet researchers have determined that, as with Panax ginseng, substances in eleutherococcus possess antiradical and antioxidant action. In one of the many experiments, nine-month old rats were divided into two groups; one group was used as the control, and the other group received a dose of the eluthero extract in their drinking water every other day for 320 days. At the point in time when half of them had died, the average life span of the control group was 680 days, while in the group receiving the eleuthero, it was 800 days—a difference of 21%. At the end of the experiment, when all the rats had died, the difference in their length of life was 80 days—10%.

Eleuthero Versus the Aging Process

Eleuthero has indicated its value in constitutional weakness and degeneration of the aging process. For example, a 73-year-old widow suffered from cold hands and feet, tiredness, and brain fag. These symptoms vanished after two one-month courses of eleuthero extract. Other cases include that of a 75-year-old man troubled by creaking joints, weak knees, exhaustion, and forgetfulness. After taking eleutherococcus for some time, he improved considerably. Many similar cases could be cited.

ELEUTHERO—WIDELY USED

With the official approval of the USSR Ministry of Health, Eleutherococcus senticosus extract is manufactured for use, and widely available to the Russian public. In addition, a cold drink called "Bodrost" (cheerfulness) contains eleuthero, and is also very popular among the Russian people.

In one of the published reports by Soviet scientists on an International Congress, eleutherococcus was included on the list of therapeutic agents which can be of interest for space medicine (e.g., to help protect Russian cosmonauts against stress, and to give them better endurance in space).

Eleutherococcus senticosus extract is currently available in the United States, and can be obtained from health food stores or herb companies.

METHODS OF USING ELEUTHERO EXTRACT

According to Soviet scientific reports, if eleuthero extract is taken in a single dose, it has a stimulant effect—an ability to make tiredness "drop off," and to increase physical endurance and mental work efficiency. Yet its stimulating action causes neither an exciting effect nor insomnia.

When a preparation of eleuthero is taken in repeated daily doses over a more or less prolonged period of time, it has a tonic action with a wide scope of therapeutic powers that increases mental and physical work capacity, and "all sorts of changes for the better." The increased vitality is noted not only during the treatment course itself, but also for some time (a month, month and a half) after the course has ended.

General Treatment Course

As a general treatment course of eleuthero extract, Soviet medics recommended the following:

Single doses—20 to 40 drops before meals, repeated two or three times a day to make the total daily dose of 80 drops. Dosage for children, a single dose: one drop per each year of age, repeated twice a day. A treatment course lasts for 25 to 30 days. Repeated courses are given at one or two week intervals, if necessary.

Dr. Brekhman states that "the preparations from eleutherococcus are non-toxic and harmless even when they are administered recurringly over a long period of time."

Note: The drops of eleuthero extract are taken in a little water.

SUMMARY

Soviet experience accumulated from years of extensive medical studies have determined the following therapeutic activity of eleutherococcus extract:

1. A first class adaptogen.

2. Has a marked stimulant and tonic action, e.g., builds zest, energy, stamina, and endurance; increases mental and physical work ability; helps combat everyday weariness; improves appetite and sleep; relieves signs of brain fag; improves mental and physical reflex action.

3. Delivers a therapeutic effect in functional nervous disturbances.

4. Has a remarkably protective effect against most types of stress.

5. Aids recovery in convalescence after illness or surgery, and builds strength in weakness and debility which often accompany chronic ailments.

6. Helpful in some cases of acne.

7. Contributes a protective effect against the dangers of radiation.

8. Improves the circulation.

9. Helpful in conditions where degeneration in the aging process is noted, e.g., forgetfulness and constitutional weakness.

10. Increases bodily resistance to disease, and has an antitoxic action in cases of some infections, auto-intoxications, various invasions, etc.

11. Helpful in the initial stages of atheroscelerosis.

12. Improves visual and hearing acuity.

13. Produces a normalizing effect, e.g., reduces a high cholesterol level; increases a low hemoglobin level; lowers increased sugar content in the blood (moderate and mild cases); normalizes low blood pressure and moderate forms of high blood pressure. Yet this action of eleuthero extract does not interfere with the normal functions of the body; that is, it does not in any way disturb normal blood pressure, normal hemoglobin level, etc.

LIST OF MAIL ORDER HERB DEALERS

Kwan Yin Herb Co., Inc.
P.O. Box 18617
Spokane, WA 99208

Nature's Herb Co.
281 Ellis St.
San Francisco, CA 94102
(Catalog 50¢)

Haussmann's Pharmacy
534-536 W. Girard Ave.
Philadelphia, PA 19123

Penn Herb Co.
603 North 2nd St.
Philadelphia, PA 19123

Golden Gate Herb Research, Inc.
P.O. Box 810
Occidental, CA 95465

Indiana Botanic Gardens, Inc.
P.O. Box 5
Hammond, IN 46325

K.D. Distributor, Ltd.
1038 S. Grand Ave.
Los Angeles, CA 90015

IN CANADA

Nu-Life Nutrition, Ltd.
871 Beatty St.
Vancouver, B.C., Canada

The Magick Roote
P.O. Box 522, Victoria Sta.
Westmount, Que., Canada

Index

C

D

E